Bewitching Bea

"Starr Morgayne's debut book, *Bewitching Beauty*, compassionately and earnestly tackles issues that are significant to the Craft and to one's personal development. Any woman (in particular) who has struggled with notions of self-acceptance and self-love will find Starr's words, rituals, and anecdotes ultimately comforting and connecting. The author greatly focuses on the notion of 'beauty,' and how this can be both applied and amplified to anyone, regardless of their age, body type, personality, or any other characteristic -- all without using chemical products, eating unnatural food, or idolizing youth. Women of all types who walk an Earth-based spiritual path are sure to be charmed by this much-needed book; this charming book emphasizes empowerment rooted directly in Mother Earth."

--Raven Digitalis, author of *Planetary Spells & Rituals, Shadow Magick Compendium & Goth Craft* and co-owner of Twigs & Brews Herbs

Bewitching Beauty by Starr Morgayne

Bewitching Beauty

Bringing out your inner Goddess, naturally

By Starr Morgayne

Bewitching Beauty by Starr Morgayne

Bewitching Beauty

Bringing out your inner Goddess, naturally

Written by Starr Morgayne

Cover Design by Dark Moon Press

Published by

Dark Moon Press

P.O. Box 11496

Fort Wayne, Indiana 46858-1496

www.DarkMoonPress.com

DarkMoon@DarkMoonPress.com

ISBN: 9781451585872

© 2010 Starr Morgayne

No part of this book may be reproduced or transmitted in any form or by any means without written permission from the author.

Dedication

This book is dedicated to all those women who have lived their lives thinking they could never be beautiful. To my teacher who taught me not only to live in harmony with nature but to be true to myself and find the strength inside. To my friend, Cindi, who gave me tons of advice, stories, help, practice and friendship as well as being one of my favorite Grammar Police. Also, to my family who have been here, supported me and loved me through everything.

Bewitching Beauty by Starr Morgayne

Disclaimer

Essential oils and herbs may be harmful and dangerous if used improperly. Allergic reactions and unpredictable sensitivities or illness may develop. I do not guarantee the effects of any 'recipes' printed within these pages. Any comments made about traditional uses of essential oils or herbs for healing purposes is not intended as medical advice, but purely as historical information. Consult a medical practitioner, certified aromatherapist, certified herbalist or other health care professional for any prolonged or serious symptoms you may have. This content is not intended to replace conventional western medical treatment. Any suggestions made and all herbs listed are not intended to diagnose, treat, cure or prevent any disease, condition or symptom. All material in this book is provided for general information purposes only and should not be considered medical advice or consultation. Always check with your personal physician when you have a question pertaining to your health and healthcare.

Bewitching Beauty by Starr Morgayne

Table of Contents

Introduction 1
Natural Beauty 9
   Everyday Dangers 15
      Recipes 20
Beauty Regimens 23
Maiden 31
   Goddesses of Maidenhood 31
   Self Esteem 34
      I Am Beautiful Ritual 37
   Peer Pressure 40
      Queen of the Nile Beauty Bath 46
      Dry Skin Acne Scrub 47
      Acne Prone Oily Skin Toner 47
      Easy Oily Skin Scrub 48
   Hair Care 51
      Vinegar Herb Dandruff Rinse 52
   Menarche 55
      The Menarche Ritual 57
      Natural Alternatives 60
   PCOS 62
   Endometriosis 64
Mother 67
   Love and Sexuality 68
      Love Thy Self Bath 69
      Come To Me Elixir 71
      Goddesses of Love, Lust and Sexuality 71
   Goddesses of Motherhood 73
      General Mother Goddesses 74
   Taking care of yourself 75
      Morning Wake Up Body Scrub 76

Trying To Conceive **79**
    Fertility Goddesses *80*

Infertility **83**
    A Child To Love Ritual.. *84*

Pregnancy **85**
    Pregnancy and Childbirth Goddesses..................................... *86*
    Stretch Marks B-Gone Pregnant Belly Oil................................ *90*

Miscarriage **92**

Varicose Veins... **93**

Taking Care of Baby **94**
    Goddesses For Infants and Children *94*
    Breastfeeding *95*
    Infant Massage... *96*

Natural Alternatives for Baby **97**
    Healing Herbal Baby Balm... *99*
    Healing Baby Powder... *101*
    Non-Mineral Baby Oil *101*
    Baby Bottom Balm *102*

Body After Pregnancy **103**

Dealing with Menstruation **106**

Keeping your looks **109**
    Exfoliating Facial/Body Scrub.. *111*
    Morning Oatmeal Facial Scrub *112*
    Simple Skin Toner *113*
    Easy Honey & Egg Moisturizer *113*

Going Gray... **114**

Hair Lightening Rinses **118**
    Lemon Water Rinse... *118*
    Lemon Chamomile Rinse... *118*

Darkening The Hair **119**
    Sage Darkening Hair Rinse *120*

Redheads **120**

Henna... **121**

Avoiding Empty Nest Syndrome **123**

Crone **127**
    Crone Goddesses *128*

Skin Care **130**
    Dry Skin *130*
    Dry Skin Mask *131*
    Wrinkles *133*
    Wrinkle Treatment *134*
    Liver Spots *134*
    Varicose Veins *135*

Menopause **136**
    The Croning Ritual *136*

Afterword **139**

Glossary of Terms **141**

Tools **145**

Ingredients **149**

Companies **179**

About the Author **181**

Bewitching Beauty by Starr Morgayne

Bewitching Beauty by Starr Morgayne

Introduction

Many of us battle self-esteem issues every day of our lives. This book is not only a resource for women of all ages but also my own exploration of my own life and how I have developed and am developing as a person. It is also an exploration of spirituality and how it pertains to our everyday lives as women. The reasons that I decided to write this book are many and varied. I have always had a love of the Earth and plants as well as animals and Nature in general. At a very young age I would sit outside in my backyard and sing to the flowers and trees and birds.

I was always curious about different plant life. My mother had a large garden where she grew many vegetables and I enjoyed helping her in the garden and smelling the vegetables as they grew.

My mother is very much a plant lover and so we had many houseplants all around. Because of this, one of my science fair projects in Junior High was studying the growth of plants and how outside stimuli affected them. One of the things that I found out is that talking to and playing music for them helped them grow immensely and to this day when I water my little lovelies I tell them how proud of them I am and how beautiful they're looking.

I grew up in a somewhat magical and kitchen witchy family. I learned that my paternal grandmother used to read tarot for her neighbors (and had an Ouija board hidden in her closet). My maternal great-grandmother, maternal grandmother and my mother were always baking things, especially during the holidays. During the winter holidays every year we would get together with my grandmother and aunts and we would bake cookies and fudge that we put into gift boxes for family and friends. We would have so many boxes to fill and it always took at least a weekend to get it all done but it was so much fun. I miss those days now but I can still remember the hectic, crowded kitchen and the smell of all those baked goodies.

My grandmother also canned foods and baked pies. A few years before she passed away I started bringing her a berry jam that I had made and canned myself for her birthday. She was diabetic so I would pick mulberries, raspberries and wild strawberries from my own backyard and create a jam using a sugar substitute (yes, I know these are not necessarily the best thing for you but I had to use something she was used to and wouldn't sneer at). I remember the way she would smile and how it would shine in her eyes when I would arrive with four jars of the stuff saying, "Happy birthday, Gramma!"

My great-grandmother used to make strawberry rhubarb pie from the rhubarb she grew in her backyard. I remember trying to read some of the old family recipes, where things were measured in pinches and handfuls, and thinking how wonderful it was. I still think of my great-grandmother as the inspiration to my own kitchen witchery.

My love of making things as well as my love of herbs and other plants grew as I got older. In my late teens I became interested in my Native American heritage. I began going to powwows and creating Native style jewelry. After a few years, I met my husband and we both began studying our heritage, his being Cherokee and mine being Lakota. We opened our own business where we made jewelry, chokers, leather goods, etc. This got me even more interested in how my ancestors lived. I began studying what foods they ate and how they healed themselves through food and natural medicines. This got me started with making teas, bath bags, salves, etc.

Thanks to our business and random chance I met up with a woman who would change my life. Her name is Patsy Clark and she is a Shawnee medicine woman, Reiki Master, teacher and all around beautiful being.

Through her teachings I learned so much more. I slept in a tipi on her property many times. I picked St. John's Wort in her meadow, helped build an arch for the gourds in her garden, scraped a deer hide to get it ready for tanning, fed chickens, watched the sun rise and the bunnies hop across the field, suffered through many a sweat lodge ceremony and loved every minute of it.

Since that time I have continued on with my study of herbs, alternative medicine, magic, spirituality, naturopathy (healing through food) and Native cultures. For a summer or two we even lived out of a tipi in our own backyard.

Because I wanted to share my love of all these things with others I opened a small store in my hometown where I sold crafts, ritual supplies, herbs and many other things. I held classes there as well as meetings for different groups. One such group was a local Pagan alliance formed by myself and some friends. Sadly, that store is no more but the dream is not over. I plan to reopen another store similar to that one sometime in the future.

My days now are spent caring for my zoo of animals, my family and creating even more salves, lotions, potions, brews, teas and anything else I can think of.

I wanted to write this book so that I can share with you, the reader, my love of everything natural as well as the knowledge I have gained throughout my time here on Mother Earth. If we all join together to teach and learn, not only can we heal ourselves but we can also help to heal the damage that has been done to our great Mother.

Since learning of the path that I am on I have witnessed many miracles. I have watched sunrises and sunsets. I have watched a hawk make its way across the sky. These are all miracles in and of themselves. During this time of learning I was told that "everything in Nature can cure everything in Nature". The explanation of this is that every plant that we have in nature has constituents in it that can help with all the illnesses that we have in nature as well. This goes for skin care too. It saddens me to see people spraying herbicides all over their lawns to kill "those horrible weeds" and then going to their local superstore and buying dandelion greens! Many of the things that we need to sustain ourselves, keep ourselves healthy and make ourselves beautiful is right in our own backyards, sometimes literally.

Historically, it is said that Cleopatra was not a woman of exceptional beauty. She was actually quite plain looking. The things about her that have made her so famous are the fact that she had self-esteem, style, grace, intelligence and the reason she was considered such a seductress is because she used natural materials such as rose petals and other common plant material to make herself look and smell good so as to help her entice the men (and power) she went after. Women back then didn't have big corporations that spat out huge amounts of cosmetics and so they had to use what was on hand. This is, in my opinion, a healthier and more harmonious way of going about things. It is also more in accordance with our own bodies and helps them work in a more natural manner.

The information contained in this book has come from many different sources too numerous to name. In all of these years I have grown, researched and learned more than I could imagine. I hope that I can encourage you to do the same.

This book is for all women no matter what stage of life they are in. We are all beautiful and we all have the power of the goddess within us. Release that power so that you can make your way in this world, in your own way.

Bewitching Beauty by Starr Morgayne

Natural Beauty

In every day of our lives we have rituals that we do. For some of us they are just mundane rituals of everyday life. For others they are more magickal. We can implement rituals for ourselves that are both of these things combined. These rituals can help us to connect to Nature and the world around us as well as connecting with the Goddess within ourselves. Each of us has a Goddess within ourselves that we can bring out in our everyday lives.

This book is about learning how we can use more natural things we have around the house to enhance our natural beauty as well as creating better habits for ourselves that will build self-esteem and confidence as well as healthy skin and body.

We will be using many common, natural ingredients to enhance skin care and health as well as make you feel beautiful inside and out. I want you to find the beauty that shines from within and let it show to everyone you meet.

You don't need a ton of make-up and fancy brand names to make yourself beautiful. It isn't about keeping up with the latest trends although it can help you to look younger. Beauty is found all around us in everything in nature. Mother Earth has given us this bounty of ingredients at our fingertips but we overlook it because of high priced advertising. Open yourself up to the gifts that we have been given.

I won't go on too long, in this section, about the issues of using store bought cosmetics but I will say that there are many chemicals within them that contribute to early signs of aging, acne, cancer and other skin issues. Our skin is the largest organ of our body and when we put chemicals on it we absorb them into our bloodstream.

There are many companies out there that boast more natural elements within their cosmetics. One of the most familiar to a large number of people is Burt's Bees[*]. I would suggest checking out some different companies at your local health food store or even online. Do some research so that you have the information for yourself. Find out what type of companies these are. Do they use organic ingredients? Are there just a few "natural" things thrown in to make things look good? Are they really Earth friendly?

---

[*] You will find contact information at the end of this book.

Look at what is important to you and then make up your own mind about which companies you would like to try. I can buy a pear in the produce section of a store and it is a completely natural ingredient BUT it has also probably been sprayed with pesticides. So you can try to buy organic produce (the preferred way of doing things) or, if that is a bit too expensive, you can take that pear home and use a good cleanser to scrub it clean. The point here is that many things are "natural" but that doesn't make it good for your body.

You can also make your own cosmetics. I know in this fast paced world we're all busy, busy, busy but if we can't take time to devote to ourselves and making ourselves healthier then how can we fully be there to support and take care of our families?

If you are buying dried herbs to use make sure to check for freshness. Even dried herbs should retain their color and some of their scent. If it looks dried up and dead then it has more than likely lost the components that make it good to use.

Making your own skin care products or cosmetics usually doesn't really take all that much time. Besides, what are a few extra minutes when you are doing something that makes you feel good, makes you healthier and gets you in touch with your spirituality? If you have a young daughter this would be a great time to spend with her and teach her how to better take care of her own skin as well as helping her to realize the beauty within herself.

Natural beauty opens many doors for us. It is often less expensive and healthier to make our own skin care products but it also lets us take more of a role in taking care of our bodies as well as getting us back in touch with Mother Nature.

If you do plan on making your own skin care products or cosmetics I would suggest either growing as much of your own as you can or buying organically grown, fresh products. Now, I know we cannot all afford to shop organic all the time. The fact that you are taking even the first step in enhancing your beauty naturally makes a big difference and don't feel guilty if you're unable to buy organically grown products.

If you are concerned about the cost of making your own skin care products I'll give you a couple of things to think about.

When you buy the ingredients to make your own skin care products you probably won't use them all up with a few batches. The best thing about these ingredients is that they can be used for other things also. You can use them in baking, craft making, cooking, natural house cleaning products and a myriad of other things. In essence you're actually saving yourself money because they have so many other uses.

Often times, buying your own ingredients is much cheaper than buying ready-made, "natural" products. I went to a local department store to compare prices. I found a popular brand of oatmeal bath on the shelf. The only ingredient listed in it was colloidal oatmeal. (Now, in layman's terms, what colloidal means is something that has very small particles and can be mixed easily in another medium.) The brand name box was $6.96 for 12 ounces. There was also a generic brand next to it that cost $4.88 for 12 ounces. This comes out to approximately $.58 per ounce for the brand name and $.41 per ounce for the generic. I then walked over to the grocery section of the store and found a container of 100% Natural Old Fashioned Oats. The cost of that container was $2.98 for 42 ounces. This comes out to $.07 an ounce! All I would need to do is take that container of Old Fashioned Oats home and grind some up in my coffee grinder, toss it in the bathtub and I would have the same thing that I would have paid over eight times more for if I bought the brand name oatmeal bath! Not to mention, I have plenty left over to have a nice hearty oatmeal breakfast in the morning.

Big conglomerates and corporations are not out to make you healthy or look pretty or anything of the sort. They are out to make money by selling you products that they have made using the cheapest means possible. Usually this is by taking small amounts of often dangerous chemicals and combining them together to give you something that they've slapped a well known brand name and celebrity's face on. Is this the type of thing that you want to pay money for?

Something you must remember when reading this book is that before using anything that you are unfamiliar with you should do research. If it's something that you apply topically (on the surface of the skin) then you'll want to do a patch test which means that you'll want to put a little on the inside of your elbow and leave it overnight to make sure that you don't have any adverse reactions to it. Also, please contact your health care practitioner before changing your diet or ingesting anything that you are not familiar with.

* * *

Everyday Dangers

As I said earlier, our skin is the largest (and one of the most important) organs our body has. Anything that we put on it or in it affects our entire body.

Many products on the market nowadays use buzz words like "Herbal", "Natural" and "Organic". The problem with most of these is the fact that the companies making these products usually have very little ingredients that are herbal, natural or organic. If there is one ingredient in the product that falls into those categories then they slap that word on the label to draw you in. Make sure to read the labels on the products you buy. This way you can stay informed and make good decisions about what you put on and in your body.

I once saw a jar of "Organic" spaghetti sauce that I thought I might like to try. I picked it up to take a look at the ingredients and was shocked to see that the only organic ingredient was the tomatoes. The rest of the ingredients were the usual thing you find in your average store bought spaghetti sauce including all the preservatives and chemicals. I picked up another brand of spaghetti sauce and, though the ingredients were not organically grown, the only ingredients it had listed were tomatoes, various vegetables, herbs, spices and other things that you would find possibly in your own kitchen at home. I prefer to grow my own vegetables and can my own sauce. My family says it tastes better than the store bought stuff anyway and I can add some magick in while I'm cooking it.

This same thing applies to shampoos, face scrubs and other skin care products that you can find on store shelves. Try not to get caught up in the hype. Make sure to read the label before buying. The further down on the ingredients list something is the less of it there is in the product. Another thing to look out for is that some skin care and hygiene products contain ingredients that are just downright scary. Did you know that some toothpaste contains asbestos? This is what is commonly used for insulation in homes. Formaldehyde (yes the stuff they use to keep dead animals in for science class) is used as a preservative in many of these products also. The problem is these ingredients are not listed in the ingredients sections under their common names. If you are unfamiliar with an ingredient I would suggest looking it up and doing some research on it to find out exactly what it is. You will find information on both sides of the argument (both for and against).

Some products use petroleum byproducts. This comes from oil, the type of oil that is used to make gasoline for our cars. Why would we want to put this on our skin? There is an easy way to get around it though. If you want to make lip balms, solid perfumes, salves or the like you can easily mix beeswax and vegetable oil to get a similar consistency to petroleum jelly. Heat the oil in a pan over low heat. When it's warm slowly put in the beeswax until the beeswax is fully melted. If you want it thinner and runnier, you use more oil. If you want it thicker, just add more beeswax. I've found that using beeswax beads is the easiest because they tend to melt quicker. I have spent time shaving a brick of beeswax and it can be very tiring and time consuming.

Another problem is antiperspirants. Even though you may find it gross, your body is made to perspire (sweat). It is your natural cooling system. The way that antiperspirants work is that they clog your sweat glands so that the sweat cannot be released. If you are unable to perspire because of using antiperspirant your lymph nodes (the filters in your body that catch toxins) can become clogged which can lead to some forms of cancer. I would rather use something that works with my body naturally to keep away the smell than get cancer. Besides, the actual perspiration isn't the real culprit anyway.

The reason that places like our underarms smell is because there are little bacteria that live in that area of our bodies and feed off of our skin cells. These bacteria release gases that cause the smell we are familiar with as body odor. Sweat itself has no smell. The warmer and wetter the area the more bacteria there are and therefore the more smell there is. The best way to avoid body odor is to keep your body cool and dry. I understand that this is not always an easy task. Another thing that you can do is use natural substances (such as baking soda) to dry out the area and natural plants (such as lavender) for their antibacterial properties.

To be honest I'm almost scared to walk through the store aisles and pick up items to look at the ingredients. You never know what you're going to find. So many products have artificial fragrances on top of everything else. When I walk down certain aisles at the store I have to be very careful because these scents can trigger asthma attacks just from walking past them on the shelves.

If you want to use perfumes or colognes but they either don't last long enough or you don't want them directly on your skin here's a little tip: Spray your clothes. The heat from your body will release the scent and it will stay on your clothes longer than your body. You could also use a diffuser necklace. These lockets come in various shapes and you put small pads in them that you put essential oils or fragrance oils on. The heat from your body, again, causes the scent to diffuse. While my best friend is taking college courses, he wears a locket with a rosemary essential oil soaked pad in it to help him remember what he is learning.

If you are reading this book then it's probably safe to say that you have at least a passing interest in using more truly natural products to maintain your beauty and health. Throughout these pages you will find information on how to make or find products that are more in tune with your body's natural functions and less harmful than the chemical laden products you find in the Health and Beauty department of your local retail store.

Recipes
Some of the recipes found in this book may include essential oils which can get to be expensive but we will try to use some of the more common, less expensive oils. Also, there are only a couple of essential oils that can be used neet (undiluted) on the skin so if you come up with your own formulas using essential oils you'll want to use a carrier oil (usually a type of vegetable oil) with it.

You will want to make small batches of most of the recipes also because without proper storage and preservatives they can go bad. There are certain ingredients that can be used as preservatives (such as benzoin, Vitamin E or grapefruit seed extract) or, if you are using carrier oils, some of them can have a very long shelf life (such as Olive Oil) while others' shelf lives may be very short. Opinions vary on the length of the shelf lives of different oils but it also depends on many things with your oil. If it smells rancid or stale, don't use it. Remember to store all herbs and oils away from heat and light to get the most life out of them possible. Dry, cool and dark is the way to go. If you are using dried herbs make sure that they have retained their natural color and smell. If they are dull and brown looking they have lost their potency. Another thing to remember when using dried herbs is that you'll usually want to replace them every 6 months or so. I have been able to keep herbs for longer than that but you always need to check the color and scent. Often times I'll use older herbs for crafts where the potency is not such a big issue.

When making skin care products you can use recycled jars (baby food jars, spaghetti sauce jars, etc.) but you will want to make sure that you have sterilized them very well. You can put them in the dishwasher or soak them in very hot, soapy water for approximately 15 minutes. This will help to keep nasty things from growing in them as well as to help get out the smell of what was previously in the jar.

Bewitching Beauty by Starr Morgayne

Beauty Regimens

Some of us have a typical morning ritual. We wake up, take a shower, brush our teeth, get dressed, have breakfast and go off to school or work. There are also the evening rituals before going to bed. Maybe you take a shower, wash your hair, wash your face and brush your teeth. We may often take these rituals for granted. This should be a time to pamper yourself, whether it is gearing yourself up for the day ahead or winding down for a relaxing night.

The next time you perform these everyday mundane rituals let's try to throw some magick in with them. You can do this by lighting a candle and saying a quick blessing, using some herbs that are specific to a goal you are trying to accomplish for the day, or anything you choose to deem magickal for yourself.

First and foremost, get enough rest. If you are not getting enough sleep your body cannot function properly and it can contribute to stress, wrinkles, bags under the eyes, etc. Now, not everyone needs eight hours of rest. Personally, I do better with seven hours of sleep whereas my husband prefers about ten hours. Do what feels best for your body.

In the morning when you wake up take a deep breath and remind yourself that this is another beautiful day that the Goddess has given us to be all that we can be.

When you go into the bathroom to take your shower remind yourself that you are not only cleansing your skin but you are also cleansing your mind, your aura and your spirit as you feel the water wash over your body. You will want to take a shower instead of a bath so that everything can just run off of you, metaphorically as well as literally. Try using an uplifting body scrub to get you ready for the day ahead of you. Make sure that, when you get out of the shower, you do not scrub your body dry with the towel. This can damage your skin, especially on the face where skin is very delicate. Always pat your body dry.

When you brush your teeth tell yourself how beautiful you are. Maybe it is the way your eyes sparkle or the way your smile lights up your face. There is always something that you can look at and see the positive aspects of.

When you pick out your clothes for the day make sure that you have clothes that are not only flattering to your body type but that also make you feel good about yourself. Pick the outfit that fits the mood you would like to have for the day.

Make sure to eat a healthy breakfast. Many of us put off breakfast because we are in such a hurry to get our day started. I know you've heard it many times but breakfast is our fuel for the day. Try to avoid sugary foods as they will just cause a roller coaster effect. Get good amounts of protein so that you will be energized and ready to face the day. Avoid caffeine if possible as it causes similar effects as the sugar.

At night, when you are home, make some time for yourself, maybe after the kids have gone to bed. You should at least try to do this once a week. Take the time to pamper yourself so that you can have a nice relaxing evening or get some well needed rest. Taking some stress off of yourself will do wonders for your health and your skin.

When you come home for the evening, or before going to bed, one of the first things you'll want to do is remove all of your makeup and oily residue from the day so that it doesn't clog up your pores and causes unsightly acne, blackheads or zits.

Have a hot, clean towel ready and a bowl or sink full of hot (but not scalding) water to dampen it with. Wrap the hot towel around your face and sit back, relax and meditate. The heat from the towel will increase the circulation in your face and allow your skin to release some of the toxins held within it. It also softens skin cells so the dead ones can be removed and opens follicles. (This would be a great time to shave some of those unsightly hairs we all get. With the follicles open the hairs will be easier to get rid of.) You can leave the towel on until it cools down. You do not want to pluck hairs though. I recently learned from a professional esthetician and electrologist that plucking hairs damages the follicle and can cause problems with hair removal.

Once you remove the towel you'll want to cleanse your skin of all those dead skin cells and toxins that you've just helped to loosen and release.

You'll want to use a facial cleanser that is made for your specific type of skin (oily, dry, combination, mature).

Apply it with a cotton pad or something soft so as not to harm the delicate skin. Don't forget your neck area.

You can also use a facial steam. The simplest way to do this is to get a bowl, a towel, some herbs and a tea kettle or clean coffee pot. You'll want to sit in a comfortable chair at a table. Place the appropriate herbs (You can go through the list at the back of this book and put together what is needed.) in the bowl and place the towel over your head. You will be making a "tent" with the towel that covers your head and the bowl so that the steam will rise up into your face bringing the essence of the herbs to your skin. When you are ready, take the boiling water and pour it over the herbs. Close your eyes and make your tent. Breathe deeply and meditate. When you are finished, gently dab your face with the towel. As stated earlier, you don't want to rub or you can damage your delicate facial skin.

For deep cleansing you can apply a face mask. These are fairly simple to make and come in different varieties. You can use a peel-off mask, mud mask, cream mask, whatever works with your skin. A peel-off mask can be made using unflavored gelatin (often found in the canning section of your local grocery store), an herbal tea or even a fruit juice (which can contain acids that gently clear dead cells from your skin). A mud mask can be made in much the same way but instead of gelatin you'll be using a type of cosmetic clay such as kaolin, betonite or French Clay. Cream masks are often made with egg whites, yogurt, and other such ingredients.

Using a toner (also known as an astringent) is good for your skin because it helps tighten the skin keeping you looking young and vibrant. It also improves the circulation and helps to control oily skin. The most common natural astringent is Witch Hazel which can be found in pretty much any pharmacy or store that contains a Health and Beauty section. When buying Witch Hazel at one of these places though you want to look for one that DOES NOT contain alcohol. You do not want to use alcohol on your skin because it can seriously dry it out and cause premature aging. Thayers brand of Witch Hazel astringents are alcohol-free and some of them also contain aloe vera, lemon, peach, lavender and rose petals. You can find their contact information in the back of this book under "Companies".

After applying your astringent you'll want to moisturize your face. Even those who have oily skin will want to do this because it helps keep your skin from being too dried out from using the astringent. Balance is valuable in everything. There are many different natural things that will help moisturize your skin. We will touch on those in later chapters.

As you perform these steps make sure that you remind yourself of your own inner and outer beauty. These are just enhancements to the beauty that you already have.

* * *

Bewitching Beauty by Starr Morgayne

Maiden

From birth until around the late twenties tends to be the time in a woman's life where the Maiden aspect of the Goddess corresponds. The Maiden represents new beginnings, childhood/youth, playfulness, adventure. Along with these things comes the stress of everyday life. The waxing moon (the New Moon becoming fuller) is good time to work with the Maiden aspect and colors that correspond with it tend to be the colors we associate with Spring or new birth; pastels in pinks, blues and yellows.

Goddesses of Maidenhood

There are a variety of Maiden goddesses. Some have similar virtues where others are somewhat different. Many of these goddesses represent springtime, youth and growing independence. Feel free to call upon these goddesses for the different aspects they may bring into your life.

Abeona ~ Abeona is a Roman Goddess who was called upon to protect children who were leaving home for the first time to explore the world. She is a goddess of outbound journeys and watched over a child's steps as well as travelers in general. She is called upon to help children become more independent.

Aphrodite ~ Aphrodite is the Greek Goddess that is the equivalent of the Roman Goddess Venus. She is the Goddess of beauty and love. The word "aphrodisiac" was derived from her name.

Artemis ~ Artemis is one of the three Greek "virgin goddesses" along with Hestia and Athena. She is a symbol of youth and independence. She was also associated with the Roman goddess Diana. Artemis was the daughter of Zeus, ruler of the Olympian gods, and Leto, a goddess of motherhood and modesty. When she was born she helped her mother birth her twin brother, Apollo. Artemis is sometimes seen as a "feminist" goddess because she was very much the "tomboy" type. When she was a small child she asked her father for a bow and arrow just like her brother's, freedom from having to dress like a lady and to be free from the distraction of love and marriage among other things. She was known as a fearless but responsible hunter. The arrows she carried in her quiver caused a painless death for the animals she hunted. She was also a protective goddess, she watched over mothers in childbirth, children and animals. She valued her freedom to roam the forests and her personal space.

Artemis was also a goddess of light and of the moon. As a moon goddess she was attributed to bringing light into the darkness. She was often depicted carrying a torch to light other's way through uncharted territory. She was self-sufficient and comfortable as a leader as well as being alone with herself. She gives strength and healing to those who need it.

Persephone ~ Persephone is another Greek Goddess. She is associated with innocence, youth, independence, growth and Springtime. She was the daughter of Demeter and Zeus (before his marriage to Hera). As the story goes, Hades, the God of the Underworld, fell in love with Persephone and kidnapped her to take her with him to his Underworld Kingdom and make her his Queen. When Persephone's mother, Demeter, became so distraught that she sent the world into eternal Winter, a deal was struck so that Persephone could return home to her mother. Before she left, Hades offered her a pomegranate. Persephone knew that if she were to eat while in the Underworld she would have to stay there forever. Persephone, having grown to love Hades and her role as Queen of the Underworld, ate seven seeds from the pomegranate. Again, a deal was struck and Persephone was allowed to return home for a few months out of the year to be with her mother but was also still able to return to her husband and the Underworld.

These are only a few of the Goddesses associated with the Maiden aspect of Womanhood. Try finding a Goddess the really speaks to you. There are many out there from countless different cultures.

* * *

Self Esteem

When I was growing up I had very low self-esteem due to being overweight and mental abuse by classmates and family members. It was not until I was in my late twenties and met a wonderful man that I began to realize the potential for beauty that I kept inside.

At a very young age, I believe I was around twelve, I wrote a story. I'm not sure where the inspiration came from but the story just flowed out of me. It involved a young woman with very low self-esteem and her loving mother. When the girl was very young she was feeling depressed and downhearted about herself. Her mother saw how sad her daughter was and came to talk to her. She told her how much she loved her and that she had a special gift for her. She gave the young girl a locket and told her that only when she was extremely depressed and facing her darkest hour should she open the locket and look inside because inside she would find the most beautiful treasure ever known. Many years later, after the girl had grown into a woman, her mother passed away and she was facing a serious depression. So many things were happening in her life and she felt so helpless and alone. She felt abandoned, unwanted and that she would never find someone to love her. It is at this time that she felt the locket heavy around her throat and remembered her mother's words of so long ago. She took it from around her neck and looked at it. She knew that it was time to look inside the locket. Slowly, she opened that locket and looked inside. What she saw brought tears to her eyes and made her heart swell with love for her mother. What she found inside that locket was a mirror and what she saw in it was truly the most beautiful treasure ever known.

As young Maidens we go through many transformations. It is our journey from childhood into womanhood. It is a time of confusing emotions, bodily changes and dealing with the world around us as our hormones go haywire.

Often times we are very awkward at this stage. Some of us deal with skin issues such as acne or Rosacea. We get oily skin and pimples or we have to get braces and wear glasses. This point in life is a perfect time to work on building self esteem.

A huge issue with young ladies in this time of their lives is self esteem, even if they have grown up with loving parents. Advertising on television, in magazines and all over give us these unrealistic images that we are brainwashed into believing are real beauty. In reality, beauty is different for every person. Each of us has something beautiful about us, whether it is our eyes, our lips, or our sense of humor.

Self-esteem is about just that, the self. It doesn't matter what others think of you. It is what you think about yourself that is most important. When you begin to love yourself then you can truly find love outside of yourself.

Confidence is a highly prized attribute in any person. With confidence in yourself you can accomplish many things that you may not have thought.

Beauty is not what we see on the covers of popular magazines. Beauty is the love that we hold within ourselves and what we do with that. We can take that beauty and project it out of ourselves and spread it into the world around us.

I Am Beautiful Ritual

When you wake up in the morning, take your shower and brush your teeth, look in the mirror and see the positive aspects of your features. Tell yourself, "I am beautiful."

As you wash your face and use your toner think of Aphrodite, Greek Goddess of Romance and Beauty or Venus, the Roman Goddess of Beauty and Love, and say:

> "Goddess of Beauty
> Let it shine in me
> Goddess of Love
> Inside myself let it be"

Part of your beauty regimen should also be to stay healthy. It is important for young people to maintain good health. Too often many young people lead very sedentary lives sitting in front of a computer or television screen. They don't eat healthy, get enough sleep or they end up falling into the trap of bad influences.

In order to maintain healthy skin, a healthy body and a healthy self image you need to get the proper nutrients so that your organs can function properly and your skin remains smooth and beautiful.

As I said earlier there is a common belief that everyone should be getting at least eight hours of sleep each night but we all know how difficult that is. Also, everyone is different. Not everyone needs a full eight hours of sleep each and every night. Some need more and some need less. It would be wise to take a look at your schedule and do your best to get as many hours as makes your body feel refreshed and ready for the day when you wake up.

Also, when you wake up in the morning you will want to stay on a schedule that allows you to cleanse away the impurities that have collected on your skin as you slept and then eat a healthy and fulfilling breakfast. By doing so you not only keep your skin healthy but you keep your entire body healthy and ready to tackle the day.

First thing when you wake up you will want to drink a full glass of water. This gets your body's system moving and boosts your metabolism which will help to give you energy throughout the day as well as to help keep off excess weight. Several of the reasons that it is suggested that we drink approximately sixty-four ounces of water a day is because we need water to live. It keeps our bodies hydrated which helps to plump our skin and keep us from looking older and leathery. It also helps to keep us from eating too much. If you drink a full glass of water (and add a little bit of lemon to it for an extra boost) before a meal it will help you to feel full faster and it will give your metabolism a kickstart so that you can digest your food easier and quicker.

Take a shower or whatever other cleansing ritual you have first thing in the morning and then off to breakfast. Try to avoid sugary cereals or other types of breakfast foods. Make sure to get a balance of proteins and starches. Fruit is important also but stay away from fruit juices that are loaded with sugar. If you must drink fruit juice try getting something that is 100% fruit juice and preferably not from concentrate. All of these suggestions start you off on the right track to a healthy, productive day.

* * *

Peer Pressure

Girls (and boys) may feel pressure from their peers at school, in extra curricular activities or just in general. This pressure may be to be popular, try drugs or alcohol, be thin or a multitude of many other things. Stay true to yourself and don't let pressure from your friends, people around you, advertisements, or anything else stop you from doing so. What is right is not always popular and what is popular is not always right.

We all experience peer pressure at some point in our lives. The friends that we choose for ourselves are, undoubtedly, going to influence our actions, thoughts and opinions. When we experience peer pressure it is usually from someone we consider a friend who has a very strong personality. Many people will go along with what this person says, thinks or does for this reason. This isn't always a bad thing. The problem with peer pressure is that it often causes us to do things that we normally wouldn't. If you are confident in yourself then you are more likely to stick with your own decisions and not be so easily influenced by others.

Don't be afraid to stand your ground if someone is trying to pressure you into something you don't feel comfortable with. Your true friends will understand and those who don't aren't your true friends. In the end you will gain respect for making your own decisions.

Have you ever heard the phrase "One is judged by the company they keep"? I cannot tell you how true this saying is. As you grow and evolve the people around you will change. The better a person you become the better quality the people that you attract can be.

We've all heard "Say No to Drugs". We've all heard about the effects they can have on your brain and your body. I can't stress enough the importance of this in a young lady. Drugs, alcohol, tobacco, all of these things do horrible things to your body inside and out. They cause wrinkles and leathery skin. I won't go on and on about how bad these things are for you because we've all heard it before but please remember everything should be done in moderation and some things shouldn't be done at all.

There are studies that show that the average size of a woman in America is 152-163 pounds. This is a far cry from the stick thin models that we see in advertisements. As long as you are healthy and happy, it doesn't matter what size you are, but don't fool yourself into believing you are healthy if you aren't. Being overweight or underweight can cause some serious issues. Either one of these factors can stop your body from functioning properly. Also, each person's body is different from the next. The ideal weight for one person may be harmful for the next; it really depends on how your body is structured.

Each of us has a Goddess within us. Whether you believe in one particular Goddess or many different Goddesses with many different aspects, we have that energy within each one of us. We are beauty, strength, love, wisdom and so much more. Believe in yourself, what you can be, what you are and know that you are a valuable part of this life.

If you are a young woman reading this book then I want you to think about something. Think about something that makes you feel good about yourself. It can be a feature you like about yourself or some other trait. It can be the fact that you are good in sports or math; anything that helps you to feel good about yourself. Take that thought and hold it close to you, right next to your heart. Let it grow and fill you up inside until you are filled with self love and pride.

This time of your life would be a good time to start your own beauty regimen. It's never too early to start taking care of your skin and body and you'll appreciate it when you're older and have great looking skin and hair.

One of the things that we focus on first and foremost is our faces. This is the first thing people see and can tell a lot about you as a person. Are you a happy, healthy person or are you a depressed person who sees no value in yourself? Your skin and hair will make a first impression as well as your smile.

You need to figure out if you have oily skin, dry skin or combination skin (a mixture of oily and dry in different areas). The section of your face known as the t-zones (the forehead, cheeks and nose) is often a problem area.

For years those of us with oily skin used rubbing alcohol in order to "clean it". Unfortunately, we now know that rubbing alcohol will dry out your skin and cause it to create even more oil which just adds to the problem. Also, drying out your skin like that contributes to premature aging.

A natural alternative to alcohol can be found at your local drug store or pharmacy. You probably have even already heard of it. Witch Hazel is great for cleaning oily skin. Most often you will find it in liquid form and you can just apply it with a cotton pad or ball. This is probably the least expensive way to go. Most of the Witch Hazel commonly found in drug stores or pharmacies is made using alcohol. Try to avoid those if possible. There are other Witch Hazel astringents, such as Thayers brand (also mentioned in the previous chapter), that are not made with alcohol and are very good for the skin.

If you have bad acne and don't mind the smell you can also use Tea Tree oil (also known as melaleuca oil). Many products now contain Tea Tree oil but I would check the ingredients to make sure that you're getting something as natural as possible. Be warned that though Tea Tree oil can be used directly on your skin it can also cause irritation.

If you are prone to blackheads, whiteheads or pimples make sure that you do not "pop" them. This causes inflammation and spreading of the bacteria that causes them in the first place. If you absolutely cannot resist the urge to do so then you'll want to use clean fingers and cleanse the area as soon as you have done so to keep it from spreading.

If you do develop pimples or "zits" one way that I have found that takes care of them quickly and painlessly is to mix a little Lavender essential oil[†] with some Epsom salts. Combine the oil and salts until the salts melt and apply it to the area. Lavender is an anti-inflammatory in addition to being antiviral and antibacterial. In no time you will find that the blemish has diminished or disappeared completely.

[†] Make sure when using essential oils that you are actually getting true pure essential oils. Some companies will try to sell essential oils combined with carrier oils and still call them essential oils or you end up just getting a fragrance oil that smells like the real thing but doesn't have the same properties. One of my favorite companies to purchase essential oils from is NOW. If you cannot find their products in your local health food store you should request that they carry them or you can go to http://www.nowfoods.com and use their store finder to find somewhere near you that carries their product.

Here are some recipes that you might like to try. By starting at a young age you will do wonders for your skin as you get older and begin to worry about things like wrinkles and crow's feet.

Queen of the Nile Beauty Bath

1 drawstring bath tea bag

Powdered Milk

Rose petals

Take a bath tea bag (or a wash cloth) and fill it with some powdered milk and rose petals. Pull the drawstring and tie it closed so that your ingredients won't fall out while you're trying to use it. Run the bag under the faucet and squish it gently with your hand until the water turns milky. Soak in this delightful bath to soften your skin and give it a lovely glow. If you'd like, you can also use the bag to gently scrub your body. You can reuse the bag a couple of times but after that you'll want to clean it out thoroughly and refill it.

The essence of roses has been used for centuries for such things as relieving depression and grief, attracting love and passion (their most common association) as well as symbolizing beauty. Some say that rose oil is one of the first essential oils documented for use. They are also associated with the Zodiac signs Taurus, Cancer, Libra and Sagittarius. It should also come as no surprise that roses are associated with the planet Venus.

Dry Skin Acne Scrub

1 drawstring bath tea bag
Old fashioned rolled oats
water

Take a bath tea bag and fill it with some rolled oats (this is the kind of oatmeal that you can find in large containers at the grocery store). Pull the drawstring and tie it closed so that your oats won't fall out while you're trying to use it. Run the bag under some warm water and squish it gently with your hand until the water turns milky. Use the drawstring bag to gently scrub your face. You can reuse the bag a couple of times but after that you'll want to clean it out thoroughly and refill it.

Acne Prone Oily Skin Toner

¼ Cup Witch Hazel liquid
10 drops Lavender Oil

5 drops Tea Tree Oil

Combine the ingredients and mix well. You can apply this with a cotton ball. You'll want to cleanse your face well before using this and even though you have oily skin you'll want to use a moisturizer afterward.

Easy Oily Skin Scrub

½ teaspoon lemon juice
1 tablespoon plain yogurt
1 tablespoon cornmeal

This recipe is great for young maidens with oily skin. First you mix together the wet ingredients (yogurt and lemon juice) and then pour in the cornmeal. Then you gently massage the mixture onto your face making sure, as always, to avoid your eye area. Don't scrub too hard because you don't want to damage your skin. Rinse off with warm water and pat dry. You'll want to follow up with a good toner.

If you feel the need to wear makeup try to get (or make) the most natural you can find as well as what is right for your skin type. Makeup can clog your pores or cause breakouts that seriously damage your skin. Also, don't forget to remove your makeup every night. Leaving it on overnight can cause even more damage.

While we're on the body I will get into the frightening subject of body odor. As I discussed earlier in the "Everyday Dangers" chapter, sweat itself has no smell. There are little bacteria that live on our skin and feed off of our skin cells. The gases they release are what we smell. Areas of the body that are warmer and wetter are where they prefer to live. This is why our underarms and other areas like this tend to smell the most. These bacteria do not like cool and dry areas so keeping those areas of your body as cool and dry as possible will help to get rid of body odor. The products that you buy at your regular grocery store can have many things in them that aren't the best for your skin. Antiperspirants can be really bad because they cause you not to sweat. Sweating is your body's natural way of cooling itself off. This can lead to clogged sweat glands which are not fun!

A few years ago I found out that I am allergic to most commercial deodorants. When I use them I break out and itch like crazy. I have gone to using Tom's of Maine deodorant which is one of the few I've found that don't give me that reaction. If you would rather make something yourself than buy a commercial product you can use something to dry out the area (such as baking soda, cornstarch, or arrowroot powder) and mix in an herb or oil that has antibacterial properties (such as lavender or tea tree). If you are using an herb you'll want to use (or get help using) a coffee grinder and grind the herb into powder form. You can then mix it with the other powder. If you're using oil you can put a few drops of the oil on a cotton ball and then seal the cotton ball in a plastic baggie with the other powder to infuse it. When your powder is finished you can use it as you would any other type of body powder. You may need to reapply it now and again depending on how much you sweat and what the weather is like.

While we're taking care of our bodies we also need to take care of our hair. Your hair can be a sign of good health as well as just an attractive asset.

* * *

Hair Care

If you have a problem with frizzy or fly away hair, instead of using manufactured serums and things, try using just a small amount of jojoba oil. You put a dollop in your palm and then rub your hands together and then through your hair. This should cut down on the frizziness and you haven't damaged your hair by covering it in smothering chemicals. Also, getting your hair trimmed about every 8 weeks will help to cut down on that. If you want to have long hair you may want to do this just as the moon begins to wax as it is said to help the hair grow faster. If you would prefer not to have your hair grow faster then you would want to cut it when the moon is waning.

We are led to believe that our hair needs to be washed every day or at least every other day. This is not true. Actually, normal shampoo strips the hair and can cause damage all on its own. Our hair needs its natural oils in order to be healthy. Washing your hair once every three to four days is much better for it.

If you rinse your hair with Apple Cider Vinegar it will help to rebalance your hair's pH balance and make it much healthier. Another healthy hair tip you might want to try is giving your hair the mayonnaise treatment about twice a month. To do this you coat your hair with mayonnaise (and make sure what you're using is actual mayonnaise and not salad dressing or something like that), comb it through with your fingers or a wide toothed comb, massage it into your scalp, cover it with a shower cap, a plastic bag or plastic wrap, wrap it in a towel and let it sit for about fifteen to twenty minutes. After that just rinse your hair thoroughly to make sure that you get every bit of the mayonnaise out. You don't want to leave some in and have it spoil in your hair. The mayonnaise acts as a moisturizer and conditioner for your hair and scalp.

If you have issues with dandruff here is a recipe that may be able to help. As always, please get an adult to help you with this.

Vinegar Herb Dandruff Rinse

2 cups water
½ cup apple cider vinegar
2 Tablespoon rosemary
2 Tablespoon sage
1 Tablespoon nettle

5 drops each tea tree oil, rosemary essential oil and lavender essential oil

Heat the water and the apple cider vinegar to just before its boiling point. Remove it from the heat and add in the herbs. Steep the herbs for approximately two hours.

When the herbs are finished steeping, strain them through a coffee filter or some cheesecloth. I like to take either my coffee filter or cheesecloth and put them in a metal strainer over a bowl. When I'm straining the herbs out then I can fold the cloth over and put gentle pressure on it to make sure I'm getting everything out. When I'm finished I can throw the whole bundle (I use natural coffee filters) into the compost bucket. It's a great way to recycle and give back to Mother Earth.

Once you have the liquid strained from the herbs you'll then add in the essential oils and stir to mix everything together. You'll want to apply this to clean, damp hair (Make sure the hair is damp and not sopping wet.) and massage it in for about two to three minutes. After the massage you'll then want to rinse with cool water.

Bewitching Beauty by Starr Morgayne

If you have oily hair you may want to try adding an egg to your hair. It sounds gross but women have been doing it for centuries and it really helps your hair. Eggs contain Vitamin E which is good for hair and skin. In order to do this you'll want to beat one egg (or if you have longer hair you might need more) and apply it to dry hair. Let it dry and then wash it out with warm water. You'll want to wash with a shampoo afterward. If you do this a couple of times a week it will remove the excess oil in your hair. If you want your hair to be shiny you can combine the egg with a teaspoon of olive oil.

To make your hair soft and shiny you can wash it in milk. Wash your hair as you normally would first. Then, wash your hair in milk and leave it on for about ten to fifteen minutes. Rinse it with warm water and you are good to go.

If you like recipes, I recently found a very interesting book at our local library. It is entitled *Beauty Trix for Cool Chix; Easy to make lotions, potions and spells to bring out a beautiful you* by Caroline Naylor. I read through it and it has some really great information as well as recipes for temporarily coloring your hair, making lip balm, and much more. It isn't exactly a magickal book but I do think it would be a good one for a young tween or teen girl.

* * *

Menarche

One of the major changes we go through that contributes to skin issues, among other things, is referred to as Menarche. Menarche is a young woman's first menstrual period. This can be an exciting and scary time for most young ladies. This is the turning point from childhood to womanhood. In times long since past this was a huge milestone for a young woman. They were pampered and made to feel good about becoming a woman.

In some Native American cultures a woman's "moon time" was a time when she was very powerful. Women were often sent to what was commonly referred to as a "moon lodge" where she sat crafting, laughing, joking and telling stories with her fellow sisters as older women who had already gone through menopause brought them extra padding for their thongs, food and anything else they might need.

In today's society we have come to view menstruation as dirty and disgusting. Women "put up" with having to deal with it every month rather than rejoicing in the natural process that makes them women. We need to take back our femininity and rejoice in it. Menstruation is not some vile thing that we have to be ashamed of. It is our body's way of saying "You are woman. You can create life." This is what makes every one of us a goddess in our own right.

Menarche is not only a time to rejoice and celebrate womanhood but it is also a time to remind yourself (or, if you are her guardian, the young lady) of your responsibilities as a woman; to respect your body and yourself. Though you are now able to have children you should know that this is a huge undertaking and you should know yourself well enough to decide when the time is right.

Here I will provide some information on Menarche rituals. These are suggestions that you can use when you decide to perform your own ritual. Not only do these rituals help young women be more comfortable with the changes happening within their bodies but they also encourage bonding between mother and daughter.

If you are a mother or guardian reading this section, make sure that the young lady is able to help with the ceremony and have as much input as possible. After all, this, for all intents and purposes, is for her. She may feel awkward about it at first and a little embarrassed but try to help her through those feelings and to feel good about what is happening to her. In many of these rituals women (meaning anyone who has already been through Menarche, including other young ladies) are the only ones present. You may hold a sort of "reception" afterwards where the males and younger girls who have not been through Menarche can congratulate the new woman if she feels comfortable with this.

The Menarche Ritual

Many Menarche rituals incorporate a lot of the color red, for obvious reasons. This can be done using clothing, candles, decorations, jewelry, or anything else you can think to use. As I said before, if you are a mother reading this section, you will want to have your daughter involved as much as possible. You can invite your/her friends that she/you feel/s comfortable sharing this special time with. Invite women who will love and support you/her. You/she can pick out some toys or one toy in particular that represent your/her childhood. If you/she choose/s many toys, these can be donated to a local charity or families in need to represent you/her moving on from childhood to womanhood. If you/she choose/s one toy you/she will symbolically give that toy up during the ritual.

An activity that everyone might enjoy is discussing the women who have touched their lives or inspired them, from relatives to celebrities. Discuss the positive aspects of being a woman as well as the responsibility involved with it.

You can start the ritual with everyone getting comfortable. Maybe you want to spread a bunch of pillows on the floor to sit on. You will then explain to everyone what the ritual is and maybe discuss the importance of these types of rituals in many cultures. As suggested before, you can tell stories of women who have been important in your lives or have the women who have been through menarche tell the young girls of their experience. You can make crafts, have snacks or any other activities that you might enjoy and that are appropriate for the occasion.

When you feel the time is right you can have all of the women stand on one side of the room and all of the young girls (who have not been through menarche) stand on the other side. You will then want to put a scarf or something representing a line on the floor separating the two groups.

The young lady being honored will then stand on the side of the line with the other young girls while holding a toy that you/she has chosen. You may then want to express your feelings as to what having the ceremony means to you. When the time comes the mother, if she is the one providing the ritual or a woman there who is important to you if you are the young lady being honored, will ask if you (or the girl the ritual is for) are ready to step beyond the threshold of childhood (this is what the toy represents) and embrace womanhood. If you/she says yes, you/she will hand the toy off to one of the other young girls and step over the line. When you/she steps over, the other women should embrace you/her and show you/her much love and affection. At the end of the ceremony, if you are the one holding the ceremony for the young lady, you may want to give her back one of the items from her childhood that she has chosen to give up and tell her that even though we grow into womanhood we still shall keep reminders of our childhood to keep us young at heart and never lose touch with the child within ourselves.

Over all, make sure that this is a happy time for the young lady so that she will not grow up to fear and loathe the natural function of her own body the way some of us have.

* * *

Natural Alternatives

There are many natural feminine hygiene product substitutes for the chemical laden products on our local grocery store shelves. There are so many dangers with using these scent-filled products, not to mention what they do to the environment. Also, by using more natural methods you can save yourself money, which is always a good thing.

For those of you who still wish to use the disposable type, you can get tampons as well as pads that are 100% natural cotton. There is a company called Natracare that produces 100% organic cotton tampons and pads (that are non-chlorine bleached) as well as sponsoring a program called Teens for Safe Cosmetics. They even do a school program to help teachers with the issues of puberty, menstruation, reproduction and environmental issues.

For those of you who may be a little more adventurous there are companies who sell reusable methods. These not only save money, because you don't have to continuously buy new products all the time, but they also help save the environment by not clogging up the landfills with products. One such company is called GladRags. GladRags sells reusable pads (you can wash them in the washing machine), menstrual cups, and sea sponge tampons.

The menstrual cups I'm referring to are made of natural materials and are inserted into the body to catch the menstrual flow instead of absorbing it. When they become full the cups are removed from the body and emptied.

Nowadays there are so many alternative ways to keep yourself healthier, help the environment and not be ashamed of your body's natural function. These products are a wonderful way to start you on your journey to womanhood.

* * *

PCOS

Although it is natural for a young lady to not be completely regular when she first starts to menstruate, if there is an issue of irregular menstrual cycles for an extended period of time there may be a problem. If there are other issues, such as hirsutism (excess body hair, especially on the face or stomach area), painful cycles (excessive cramping to the point of being debilitating), extremely heavy cycles, no cycles at all, weight gain in the stomach area, thinning hair or areas of the skin that appear dirty no matter how many times they are washed, this may be a sign of a hormonal imbalance known as Polycystic Ovary Syndrome (also known as PCOS). This is a problem that is growing rapidly in our society. If you or someone you know presents with these problems please get checked or encourage them to get checked. Another of the symptoms of this condition is infertility. If caught early you may be able to do a lot more to help your body get back on track.

In the past many doctors have chosen to treat this problem by prescribing birth control pills. This may compound the problem as birth control pills are synthetic hormones (usually estrogen or progestin) and this problem is already caused by hormones being out of whack. We live in a society where women (as well as men) are starting to become estrogen dominant due to the fact that the animals we eat are pumped full of hormones to make them bigger so that more money can be made off of them. This is just contributing to the problem.

PCOS is also linked to Diabetes (especially Type 2 Diabetes) or Insulin Resistance as they are all metabolic disorders and can develop into a nasty catch 22 situation. By catching it early and treating it properly you may be able to save yourself and the ones you love a great deal of heartache and pain.

If you have a daughter or loved one with these problems they may be too embarrassed by it to talk about it. If it goes untreated it can cause many other problems (such as the infertility and Diabetes I spoke of).

When I was a young girl I had many of these issues but since doctors have only gained a slight bit of knowledge about PCOS in the last generation I was told that my problems were caused by many other things. I was put on birth control pills, made to start a food diary and harassed by a doctor who didn't know what was wrong with me. I was continually accused of lying in my food diary because he didn't believe I could eat as little as I did and still weigh as much as I did.

When, in my early 20's, we found out what the real problem was, my mother came to me with tears in her eyes apologizing for everything I had been put through because she didn't know any better.

To this day I am still dealing with PCOS and trying to treat it as naturally as I possibly can. I take several pills a day (things like Evening Primrose Oil, Chaste Tree Berry {also known as Vitex}, and Red Raspberry Leaves) and try to eat foods that will not only help me lose weight but also help to balance my hormones.

* * *

Endometriosis

Endometriosis is a condition in which the cells (called endometrial cells) inside the uterus grow outside of the uterus. It is mainly affected by hormones, similar to PCOS. Some more noticeable symptoms of Endometriosis are pain in the pelvic area or lower back, irregular bleeding, painful periods, possible infertility. Sometimes there are no symptoms at all.

Both Endometriosis and Polycystic Ovary Syndrome can be mild to severe and have similar symptoms. Some doctors will say that the best option for treatment is a hysterectomy. A hysterectomy is an operation in which the doctor removes a woman's uterus. The uterus is where a baby grows when a woman is pregnant. Sometimes, the rest of the reproductive organs are also removed. This includes the ovaries (which make a woman's eggs and hormones) and the fallopian tubes (which carry the eggs from the ovaries into the uterus to be fertilized).

When I was being treated for PCOS by a fertility doctor this was recommended to me. Because I wanted to have children, I decided not to go through with it. I wanted to do whatever I could to try to fix my body to the best of my ability so that one day I might be able to have children of my own.

If you are having some of these issues you might want to speak to someone about it so that it doesn't cause even more problems in the future.

* * *

As we grow out of the Maiden stage we come to the Mother stage. This is a time in our lives when we really experience womanhood and the joys and frustrations that go with it. Going from the Maiden stage to the Mother stage of life can be a painful but enlightening journey. As you'll see in the next chapter, Motherhood is not just about having children. It is about realizing your full potential and power within yourself. It is about using the power of the Goddess in you to push yourself toward your goals. It is about nurturing that which is inside you to fruition.

Mother

The Mother aspect of the goddess seems to be the most popular. That could be because we often focus on the Goddess as our mother along our path. She helps to guide us on our journey, console us when we're grieving and lift us up when we're down. You need not have children to realize the Mother aspect of the Goddess within yourself. Some mothers that don't have human children look to their pets as their, what are sometimes called, "fur children". I know that the animals I have in my life mean as much to me as the little people running around my home. Creation is what the Mother is about. Crafting, creating a business, nurturing a garden, these are all Mother types of activities.

This time of our life is about nurturing (of ourselves and others), caring, unity and fertility. These can represent many things. This is a time to nurture ourselves, our dreams, our goals and our loved ones. It is a time for unity with other Gods and Goddesses within others and fertility of not only the body but the mind and the efforts we make for ourselves. A woman is at the peak of her power during this period of her life. The Mother is life; the source of all creation. Whether that is creation of another human life or the creation of an idea is to be realized by you.

* * *

Love and Sexuality

We all need and feel love in one form or another. At this point in our lives (when we are heading out of the Maiden phase) love can weigh heavily on our minds as we think of finding a life partner and possibly getting married or raising a family.

In order to love another and to be loved back we must first learn to love ourselves. That is one of the reasons for my writing this book. We, as women, must love ourselves and pamper ourselves now and then in order to maintain a healthy mind, body and spirit. In return, we may also find that we have self-confidence (which is very sexy) and that we can become self-reliant as well. We can be self-assured and sexy at any age and shape. They say that beauty is in the eye of the beholder and what beholder is more important than yourself? Let your inner Goddess shine through for all to see, whether that Goddess is Lilith (a sexy succubus) or Gaia (the earth mother). Don't be afraid to switch things up a bit now and then either. It's a woman's prerogative to change her mind often.

Love Spells are often the most sought out spells. Many say that you should not use a love spell on a specific person. There is wisdom behind this warning. You've heard the old saying "Be careful what you wish for". This is the issue with love spells that have a certain target. How do you know that this person is that absolutely right person for you? If you decide that you want to perform a love spell I would suggest performing a more generalized love spell. One that brings love into your life in whatever form it appears. Whether you prefer to call it cause and effect, karma, the rule of three or any similar thing, the energy you put out does come back to you. We must remember that everyone has free will and to tamper with that can mess things up in a seriously bad way.

Love Thy Self Bath

Candles (pink for love, red for positive thinking, orange for strength, yellow for self confidence)

Rose petals (love)

Before you get into the bath take a shower and wash off in order to cleanse yourself of all negative energies and influences.

Run a bath with water hot enough to be relaxing but not hot enough to scald you. Light your candles and sprinkle the rose petals in the bath or tie them up in a washcloth or bath bag and drop them in the water. Slowly sink into the bath, put a folded towel under your neck and lay back and relax. Think about all of the positive aspects of yourself.

When you're finished with your bath and you step out of the tub to dry off make sure that you have some nice lotion to put on your skin. Hot water dries the skin out and by adding a good humectant lotion you can help to keep your skin silky, smooth and sexy.

When you're ready to go out looking for love (or lust) there are many things that you can do to get yourself "in the mood".

The following recipe is one of attraction. It uses compelling herbs and spices combined with those for love.

Come To Me Elixir

1/8 teaspoon cardamom (love and lust)

½ teaspoon allspice (luck)

½ teaspoon orange peel (love)

1 teaspoon cloves (love)

1 cinnamon stick (lust, love and power)

1 cup apple cider (love)

This recipe is great for a cool fall night when you want to feel seductive. Combine the cardamom, allspice, cloves, and orange peel in a tea bag or cheesecloth. Heat the cup of apple cider and steep the herbs in it for a few minutes. Use the cinnamon stick to stir the apple cider and sip as you think sexy thoughts. If you like you can substitute red wine for the apple cider.

Goddesses of Love, Lust and Sexuality

Freya ~ Freya is a Norse goddess. She is a warrior goddess, a Valkyrie, as well as a goddess of sensual love and sexuality.

Aphrodite ~ Aphrodite is the Greek Goddess that is the equivalent of the Roman Goddess Venus. She is the

Goddess of beauty and love. The word "aphrodisiac" was derived from her name.

Lilith ~ The Sumerian Goddess Lilith was also known as a Succubus. Succubi were often looked upon as demons who "stole men's seed" as they slept. She is a powerful goddess to work with when it comes to seduction, sensuality and sexuality.

You can feel sexy just by wearing something slinky under your normal everyday clothes. Who cares whether or not anyone else will see it? This is about you and how it makes you feel. Sexy doesn't have to be slutty or low class either. You can wear a nice classy outfit and feel just as sexy. Pick out what works best for you. Build your confidence.

When you're feeling sexy and confident, make your move. Sometimes it's just nice to go out and get some attention, a little flirting, or maybe find the someone you've been looking for. You are in control of your own destiny. Make of it what you will.

* * *

Goddesses of Motherhood

Many of the Mother Goddesses we find represent home and hearth. This is not because of an antiquated idea that a woman should be at home in the kitchen but, oftentimes, because the home and hearth were the most important places in ancient times. The women would "keep the home fires burning", literally. While the men were out hunting the women kept their home running smoothly so that the men would have something to come back to. They would keep the hearth or "home fire" burning so that they would have heat, light and be able to cook meals throughout the day. They took care of the children, the home and the food. Women are the life blood of society. In my opinion I think we have lost some of that because we've become so focused on trying to get past patriarchal conditioning that we've lost our own sense of purpose.

As I've said before, women were most important to many ancient civilizations. We were not only the givers of life but we were the decision makers. We appointed leadership roles. We hunted alongside the men. We have played every role imaginable. Now is the time to realize the potential you hold within yourself as a woman. You can be strong as well as sexy. You can be smart *and* beautiful. You can be vulnerable yet in command.

The Mother aspect of the Goddess represents healing, sexuality, love, growth, abundance. The Full Moon is a good time to work with Mother Goddess energy.

There are a number of Mother Goddesses. As with the Maiden goddesses, some have similar virtues where others are somewhat different. There are goddesses for fertility, pregnancy, childbirth, protection of the hearth and home, many aspects of motherhood. Feel free to call upon these goddesses for the different aspects they may bring into your life.

General Mother Goddesses

Aka ~ Aka was an Ancient Turkish Mother Goddess

Ceres ~ Ceres is the Roman Goddess of farming, crops and agriculture. She is the Roman equivalent to the Greek Goddess Demeter. She was also a goddess of motherly love.

Demeter ~ Demeter was the Greek Goddess of the Harvest and of the Fields. She was the devoted mother of Persephone.

Gaia ~ Gaia is the ancient Greek mother goddess who gave birth to the land as well as the Titans. She is the earth and the creator.

Hestia ~ Hestia is the Greek counterpart to the Roman Vesta. She is the Goddess of hearth and home. She was the first born of the Olympian gods.

Uma ~ Uma is an Eastern Indian Goddess. Uma means "light". She is the power that stands hand in hand with the God.

* * *

Taking care of yourself

As we step from Maidenhood into Motherhood things will change drastically but that doesn't mean you have to let yourself go. As a mother you will need to pamper yourself even more to combat the new stressors in your everyday life. You have the responsibility of taking care of so many other things but, as I have been told repeatedly by my loved ones, how can you take care of everyone else if you don't take care of yourself first and foremost?

Here is a recipe for the busy mother on the go. It is great to use in the shower first thing in the morning.

Morning Wake Up Body Scrub

1 cup Coffee Beans (can be Peppermint flavored)

¼ cup salt

3 tablespoons extra virgin olive oil

3 drops vitamin E oil

2 drops peppermint oil

You can make this at any time and then store it for later use. It should last for quite a while. Don't worry if it dries out after a time. The coffee beans will soak up the oil but it still works just as well. The first step you will want to do is to grind your coffee (if it is in bean form) into very fine granules. After that combine all of the ingredients and stir well. You will want to use this in the shower because if you try to use it in a bath it will get very messy.

Take a small scoop of the scrub and use it to scrub your entire body except for your face. The coffee is too harsh to use on the face. It might feel a little different at first. That is probably the extra virgin olive oil coating your skin. Rinse thoroughly. After you finish your entire shower you may have to rinse out the bottom of the tub or shower stall to get all of the scrub down the drain.

I was inspired to create this recipe by a walk through our grocery store one day. I love walking through the coffee aisle and smelling the coffee beans. During the holidays we went for a stroll down the coffee aisle and I smelled this enchanting aroma. It was a peppermint flavored coffee only put out for the holidays. The idea suddenly struck me. Coffee and peppermint are both things that wake you up and exhilarate you! So, I grabbed a pound of coffee beans and brought them home to formulate my scrub.

I often use my friends as test subjects for my concoctions but I haven't had any complaints yet. One such friend recently started working two jobs, one being third shift. She also has a family to take care of during the day. Her first week on the job was very hard on her and she barely slept for a few hours each day. I gave her some of this scrub to try. The next day she called me and couldn't wait to tell me about it. She told me about how all day she had been a walking zombie and had even dozed off during the last bit of a class she was taking. When she came home she decided to try out the scrub. Standing in the shower, as she washed her hair and did her usual rituals, she was still falling asleep. Then she reached for my scrub. She said the minute she started using it she was like WOW! She told me that it immediately woke her up and she absolutely loved it!

This recipe has many different benefits, besides waking you up of course. The coffee beans used as a scrub are not only exfoliant but the caffeine within them helps to get rid of cellulite. The salt is another common exfoliant used in many body scrubs. The extra virgin olive oil is a humectant that draws and holds moisture to the skin. My friend said that after she used it her skin felt absolutely heavenly. We all know that Vitamin E is good for keeping the skin soft and healthy and the peppermint oil is good for waking up the senses. By using this not only will you be pampering your skin but you will also give yourself a head start on those early mornings when the kids are already up and roaring to go.

You can also use variations of this recipe. For a coffee scrub that is decadent and seductive try using Chocolate

Almond or French Vanilla flavored coffee and leave out the peppermint oil. Another you can try is using Hazelnut flavored coffee. Hazelnuts are associated with judgment and wisdom.

* * *

Trying To Conceive

Fertility Goddesses tend to be the most popular of all of the aspects of the Goddess. Archeologists have found some of the earliest Goddess images were of the pregnant Mother Goddess with her swollen belly and large breasts. This represents the fertility of people, animals and the land we live on. Many moon goddesses are associated with fertility due to the fact that a woman's menstrual cycle often followed the waxing and waning of the moon and women tended to be more fertile during the time of the full moon.

It is not uncommon for couples to place a statue or representation of fertility gods or goddesses on a family altar or near their bed along with an offering to the deity to insure their own fertility or at least help it along.

Here is a list of some goddesses that have been associated with fertility:

Fertility Goddesses

Ala ~ Ala is a goddess of the African people of eastern Nigeria. She is considered a mother goddess of the earth, guardian of the harvest, ruler of the underworld and goddess of fertility for both people and animals. It is believed that she makes the child grow within its mother's womb.

Bast ~ Bast (also known as Bastet) is a well known Egyptian goddess that is associated with both fertility and childbirth. She is most often portrayed as a slender woman with the head of a cat and was the daughter of Ra (Osiris) and Isis. She was a goddess of many things, one of them being the protector of the household. The feline essence is often seen as the ultimate in feminine sexuality and Bast also represents this as well as the mother cat and her litter of kittens, corresponding with fertility.

Bendis ~ Bendis was a Greek moon goddess and that is where her association with fertility comes from. She was very similar to Artemis.

Bona Dea ~ Bona Dea was the Roman goddess of healing, virginity and fertility in women. She was known as "the good goddess". She was the daughter of the god Faunus and was often referred to as Fauna. She healed the sick in her temple garden with medicinal herbs.

Cybele ~ Cybele is a Phrygian goddess who was very similar to Gaia in that she is the "Mother of All" also known as the "Mountain Mother".

Frigg ~ Frigg is a Norse Goddess who was married to Odin. She is a goddess of marriage, childbirth, motherhood, wisdom, household management and weaving and spinning. Barren women would invoke her and ask her to bless them with children.

Gaia ~ Gaia is the ancient Greek mother goddess who gave birth to the land as well as the Titans. She is the earth and the creator. She is often shown as a woman whose belly looks pregnant and is colored like the earth.

If you are in the process of trying to conceive you need to make sure that both you and the prospective father (if he is actively involved) are taking the best possible care of your bodies that you can. Make sure that you are maintaining or trying to reach a good weight and that you are practicing healthy lifestyle habits to achieve a good environment to produce a little one. Make sure that you are getting enough vitamins that are needed to maintain a healthy pregnancy even before you conceive. You can even start taking prenatal vitamins ahead of time to help your body get ready to carry a baby.

Red raspberry leaves and Vitex (chaste tree berries) are a couple of the herbs that are commonly known to help with female hormone and reproductive issues. Nettle has many nutrients that are helpful to expecting mothers or those who would like to be. Rosemary Gladstar and Susun S. Weed have some great information and recipes in their books *Herbal Healing for Women* (Rosemary Gladstar) and *Wise Woman Herbal for the Childbearing Year* (Susun S. Weed). You might also want to check out Jeanne Rose's *Herbs & Aromatherapy for the Reproductive System*.

Pay attention to your menstrual cycle (or moon cycle as it is sometimes called) and learn how to chart your fertility through natural means. This can help if you want to become pregnant or even if you want to try to avoid pregnancy right now. Knowing our bodies better is never a bad thing.

If you are having difficulty in conceiving you will probably be receiving all kinds of advice from well meaning family members, friends, strangers, etc. Don't let this frustrate you. Most of all do not let the stress of trying to conceive or infertility get you down. Stress is so hard on our bodies and will just make the process that much more difficult. My husband and I received all kinds of advice while we were trying to conceive; from if we just stopped trying it would happen to "get drunk and then try, that's what we did!"

Though the advice is well meant it can be extremely hard to deal with because most people don't understand the stress and heartache that go into trying to conceive. It comes so easy to some while others struggle for years and may never achieve the pregnancy they so long for.

Infertility

If you have been having unprotected sex for more than a year and have not conceived that is considered infertility. There may be a simple fix for this or it may be more complicated. Make sure to check with a health care professional first and foremost to see what might be the problem. Also, if you have a male partner, never assume the problem is solely with you. You both should get checked out so that you know exactly what the issue is and can deal with it together. To help out you can also check in the Ingredients section of this book and find items that are magickally inclined to fertility.

Here is a spell that you can try:

A Child To Love Ritual

Gather together herbs representing fertility. If you are focusing on wanting a girl get together a pink candle and herbs representing femininity. If you are focusing on wanting a boy gather together a blue candle and herbs representing masculinity. If you don't mind which sex the child will be then I would suggest the use of a white candle. If you like you can burn the herbs in a cauldron (representing the womb) but make sure that the herbs you have gathered are safe to burn and that you have adequate ventilation.

When you are ready, light the candle and gather the herbs together while you infuse them with your energy and focus your intent. If you plan on burning them you can then sprinkle them over a charcoal briquette in your cauldron as you chant these words:

Mother Goddess hear my plea
Bring a child to my family
My special gift to cherish and love
It is all that I can think of

To hold them in my arms
And keep them safe and warm
To feel them growing inside my belly
As I will, so mote it be

There are quite a few books on fertility that you can check into also. Two books that I hear talked about most often are *Wise Woman's Herbal For the Childbearing Years* by Susan S. Weed and *Taking Charge of Your Fertility* by Toni Weschler.

* * *

Pregnancy

Pregnancy is a joyous occasion for many but also a very scary time even if the pregnancy was planned. Here are some goddesses that may help you get through this chaotic time:

Pregnancy and Childbirth Goddesses

Artemis ~ Artemis was the twin sister of Apollo. When she was born she immediately played the role of Midwife to her mother who was having difficulty delivering her brother. Because of this she has been associated with childbirth and labor. Women would call upon her to ease the birth and the labor pains of their delivery.

Aveta ~ Aveta was a Gaulish goddess associated with midwifery and childbirth.

Candelifera ~ Candelifera was a Roman goddess that was usually invoked at the beginning of childbirth. She was the candle barrier and lit the way to help guide the baby into the world.

Hecate ~ Hecate was, amongst other things, a Greek goddess of childbirth. She carried a sacred knife on her so that she could cut the umbilical cord of the child she was delivering.

Lucina ~ Lucina was a goddess of childbirth in Roman Mythology. She guarded the lives of women in labor.

Meshkhenet ~ Meshkhenet was an Egyptian goddess who represented one of the bricks where women in ancient

Egypt stood in a squatting position to give birth. She is often seen as a brick with a female head. Not only did she ensure the safe delivery of the baby but she also decided the child's destiny as soon as they arrived in this world.

Nintur ~ The Sumerian Goddess Nintur was a creation Goddess, a Mother Goddess and Goddess of the womb.

Rumina ~ Rumina is a Roman Goddess of Breastfeeding. She causes milk to flow.

Nona ~ Nona is the Roman Goddess of Pregnancy.

Prorsa Postverta ~ This Roman Goddess was the Goddess of women in labor and was associated with the child's position within the womb.

There are a few herbs that should be avoided during pregnancy so make sure to check into these so that you don't accidentally use something that could be harmful to you or your baby. Some of these herbs, such as pennyroyal, can cause miscarriage. Here are some other herbs that you may want to avoid: Angelica, Anise, Arnica, Ashwaganda, Barberry, Basil, Bitter Melon, Black Cohosh or Blue Cohosh (except during last few weeks of pregnancy), Blessed Thistle, Borage, Camphor, Caraway Seeds, Castor oil, Catnip, Celery Seeds, Cinnamon, Comfrey, Dong Quai, Echinacea, Elecampane, Ephedra, False Unicorn, Fenugreek, Feverfew, Ginger, Goldenseal, Guarana, Honeysuckle, Horehound, fresh Horseradish, Horsetail, Hyssop, Juniper, Lemongrass, Licorice, Lobelia, Lovage, Marjoram, Mistletoe, Motherwort, Mugwort, Myrrh, Nutmeg, Oregon Grape Root, Parsley, Pennyroyal, Pleurisy Root, Poke, Prickly Ash, Red Clover, Rosemary, Rue, Saffron, Sage, Sassafras, Sarsaparilla, Savory, Saw Palmetto, Shepherds Purse, Spikenard, St. John's Wort, Tansy, Tarragon, Thyme, Turkey Rhubarb, Turmeric, Uva Ursi, Vitex (Chaste Tree), Watercress, White Sage, Wormwood, Yarrow and Yucca. This is by no means a complete listing and you should **always** check with your health care practitioner before ingesting any herb during pregnancy.

Red raspberry leaves have been used for centuries to tone the uterus during pregnancy and this is one of the herbs that are actually sometimes recommended during pregnancy.

Nettle is another herb that has been recommended during pregnancy because it provides some wonderful nourishment and helps to prevent blood loss after the birth.

Peppermint, Catnip, Chamomile and Ginger are often recommended to those women suffering with morning sickness. Drinking these herbs in tea form can help in more than one way. By sitting and relaxing with a cup of tea you are also relieving some of the stress from you and the baby.

One of the first things that most new mothers-to-be worry about is stretch marks. Some women are proud of their stretch marks and wear them as a badge of honor. There is absolutely not a thing wrong with this. I commend these women but there are also those women who would rather not have them. There is nothing wrong with that either. There are many things you can do to help your body cope with its changing shape. It is a common misconception that all expectant mothers need to gain weight. That is not necessarily true. Speak with your health care practitioner on whether or not you need to gain, lose or maintain the weight you are currently at.

Regardless of whether you will be losing, gaining or staying the same weight your skin is going to stretch to accommodate the little life you are carrying inside. Here is a recipe you can try that you can massage onto your growing belly (or have a special loved one massage it on for you) to help keep the skin elastic and minimize your stretch marks.

Stretch Marks B-Gone Pregnant Belly Oil

½ cup extra virgin olive oil

6 vitamin E capsules (or ½ tablespoon vitamin E oil)

¼ cup aloe vera juice

4 vitamin A capsules

2 drops Benzoin

10 drops Lavender

Blend all ingredients together until emulsified (where everything is blended together completely). Store in refrigerator. Shake well before using. Apply liberally and rub in.

Also in the Natural Alternatives for Baby[‡] section you will find recipes for your new baby when it arrives. If you're not an expectant mother but you know of one these might be great to make up as gifts to give at a baby shower.

[‡] Page 97

Pregnancy can be a trying time with morning sickness, chaotic hormones and worrying about the baby as well as all the other fun things that go with it. Make sure to relax and take care of yourself and focus on what you are accomplishing. You are bringing forth another life. Find pictures or statues of the pregnant goddess to meditate on and give you strength. Try to stay as relaxed and stress free as possible as this will be better for you as well as for the baby.

During pregnancy, because your body's hormones are changing, it can also change your skin. You can go from oily to dry, dry to oily or anything in between. The skin care products that you used before your pregnancy may not work properly for you during pregnancy.

Make sure that you keep an eye on your skin so that you know when and if these changes occur. By doing so you will be able to tailor your skin care products to what your skin needs during that time.

When time gets close for you to have your baby, if you plan on having the baby naturally, I have a tip I can offer. When I was studying midwifery for a short time it was recommended that you (or, more than likely, have a partner) massage the perineum (the area between the vaginal opening and the anus) with some vegetable oil (such as olive oil) in order to relax the muscles in that area to prevent tearing or the need for an episiotomy (where the doctor cuts you just a little to help get the baby through and prevent or minimize tearing).

Miscarriage

Miscarriage is a terrible but often very real reality for many of us. It is a scary and heartbreaking time. It can also be very dangerous. If you suspect you are having a miscarriage, please, contact your health care practitioner. If you are at risk for miscarriage please discuss that with your health care practitioner as well.

As said previously, avoid certain herbs that may contribute to miscarriage. See the list starting on page 87 for some of the herbs to avoid.

There are steps you can take to help reduce the possibility of miscarriage but often times there is just nothing you can do to completely prevent it. Make sure to follow your health care practitioner's advice, eat healthy and try not to stress because stress can help to cause a miscarriage also.

Vitamin E, Wild Yam Root and Red Raspberry Leaves are all said to help prevent miscarriages from happening.

Varicose Veins

These are often times a hazard of pregnancy. Some of the things that can help you avoid these are exercises (if you have your health care practitioners' ok) in which you lie on your back and prop up your legs for 15 minutes, swimming or walking. Yoga is also wonderful for pregnancy in so many ways. It helps the body function properly, increases circulation and you can use different postures to help different problems. Massage will help as well and massage during pregnancy has the benefits of relaxing the mother and the baby at the same time.

A problem that often goes along with pregnancy and varicose veins is hemorrhoids. Varicose veins and hemorrhoids are caused by the same issue; constriction of the blood vessels and bad circulation. Hemorrhoids can often be helped by sitting in a sitz bath made from a yarrow tea as it is anti-inflammatory and also helps to slow bleeding.

* * *

Taking Care of Baby

As we watch over our babies many of us would like to know that our Goddess/es are also watching over them. Here is a list of Goddesses that are especially good for infants and children.

Goddesses For Infants and Children

Caireen ~ The Irish Goddess Caireen is a patron Goddess of children and a protective mother Goddess.

Cuba ~ Cuba is a Roman Goddess of infants and children who watches over and blesses them as they sleep.

Renenet ~ Renenet, who was sometimes known as Renenutet, is an Egyptian Goddess who gave each infant their true soul name and presided over breastfeeding.

Edusa ~ Edusa is the Roman Goddess of weaning who would watch over infants and protect them as they transitioned from breastfeeding to eating solid foods.

Levana ~ Levana is a Roman Goddess of newborns. Her name means "the lifter" this relates to the ritual of the mother placing the child on the ground and the father lifting the baby to show that he accepted it as his own.

Lilith ~ Lilith is a Sumerian Goddess who fiercely protected mothers and especially children. Because of this, she is a good Goddess to work with for single parents.

After the birth of your baby you are going to have lots to do but taking care of your baby doesn't have to mean you let yourself go. There are many things that you can do that are beneficial to both you and baby. Some examples of this would be relaxing with some soft music, breastfeeding or infant massage. This is a good time to create those bonds with your baby that will last both of you your entire lifetimes. There is nothing like the bond between a mother and her child.

Breastfeeding

Breastfeeding is a wonderful time to bond with your baby and helps to prevent postpartum depression by encouraging your hormones to get back to a more normal state.

There are certain herbs that you can use during breastfeeding that will help with different issues also. For example, you can use Comfrey, Nettle, Alfalfa, Red Clover, Blessed Thistle, Borage, Fennel or Anise to encourage milk flow, Marshmallow Root to strengthen the milk or Sage to dry the milk up. Some foods that will help to increase and sustain milk flow are apricots, asparagus, green beans and carrots.

You'll want to massage the breasts with oil in order to keep them soft and to help bring them back into shape after breastfeeding is over. Oil infused with Calendula and Vitamin E is a good choice for this. Calendula and Vitamin E will help to keep the area soft and prevent dry, cracked skin.

Infant Massage

Infant massage is another good way of bonding with your baby. It will help to increase their circulation, relax both you and baby, and has many other benefits. Make sure to research this in order to know how to do it properly so as not to harm the baby.

You can even make your own oils to massage your baby with but you must remember to not use more than 3 drops total of any essential oils to 1 teaspoon of carrier oil when making massage oil for baby. Also, check into which oils are best used for what and which oils to avoid. Another thing you might want to remember is it is often advised not to use essential oils on babies that are less than 6 months old.

* * *

Natural Alternatives for Baby

If you are concerned about yourself and the things that you put on your own skin then it makes sense that you would be concerned about what you put on your baby's skin too. Just as we discussed in the Maiden chapter, there are natural alternatives to chemical laden diapers and other products that are used every day. The recipes you have previously read can be good alternatives to what we might find on store shelves.

Companies such as Natracare (one of the companies sited in the previous chapter), Earth Mama Angel Baby, Our Natural Baby, and many others have natural products for baby and you. My suggestion would be to research some of these companies to find out which one you would like to use and what is most affordable to you.

There are even some companies that are run solely by WAHMs (Work At Home Mothers) if you are more inclined to shop with them.

You can find many websites that will teach you how to use nappies (cloth diapers) and several other natural alternative products. Nappies are more economical and ecological than most of the diapers we see on store shelves. You don't have to purchase cloth diapers either. If you're handy with a needle and thread or sewing machine you can always make your own. I find this a lot of fun because I love going to the fabric store to pick out cute designs.

Below are some recipes that you can use that might help you to feel better about what you are putting on your baby's skin. For me there is no greater satisfaction than using something I've made myself, especially for someone so precious to me. When I make my own skin care products I can put love and good energy into them. Factories that mass produce everything aren't able to do that.

Healing Herbal Baby Balm

All three of the herbs used in this salve have been shown to be powerful yet gentle. Because of this, the salve can be used to help with diaper rash or act as a moisturizer for very dry skin. It can even help with small cuts and scratches.

2 cups extra virgin olive oil (or almond oil)
1/3 cup Comfrey
1/3 cup Chamomile
1/3 cup Lavender
6 capsules vitamin E (or ½ Tablespoon vitamin E oil)
Enough beeswax to make the salve the right consistency

Combine the herbs and oil in a saucepan or slow cooker. If you have the same trouble I do, which is using too much heat and cooking the herbs, you can use a double boiler. You don't want to actually cook the herbs. You want to heat the oil enough to infuse the herbs but you don't want to fry them. Place whatever you are using on the lowest heat setting possible. Let the herbs infuse for about 3 hours but keep an eye on them to make sure the heat is not too high. When they are thoroughly infused remove them from the heat and allow the infusion to cool off. Once it's cool you can strain out the herbs. At this time you can add in the Vitamin E oil. Now, you'll want to put the oil back on a very slight heat, just enough to warm it up and slowly add in the beeswax until it is completely melted. You can then pour the salve into your prepared containers and let it sit to solidify. If you've used too little beeswax you can warm it up again and add a little more. If you've found you've used too much beeswax then just make up a bit more oil, heat up the salve and add some of the new batch of oil to it. You may have to experiment with this a couple of times to get it precise.

If you have the time and want to infuse oil to use later you can always use an old jar (make sure the jar and lid are clean and sterile) to infuse your herbs on a sunny windowsill. This takes about two weeks of sunny weather. You place the herbs into the jar and then pour whichever oil you are using over the top. Make sure that the oil covers the tops of the herbs as this will help to keep away mold and germs. Once the oil is thoroughly infused you can then strain it out, compost the herbs and use the oil or, if you would like to make a stronger concentration of oil, you can empty the jar, put new herbs in and add the already infused oil to them. You can continue this process until the oil is as concentrated as you would like. You can use these methods with any of the recipes contained in this book that call for infusing oils with herbs. If you want to add a natural preservative you can use some Vitamin E oil or some Grapefruit Seed Extract. You should only need a very small amount of either.

Healing Baby Powder

If you want to avoid using talc on your baby you can easily make your own baby powder by combining equal parts Baking Soda, Cornstarch and Arrowroot Powder. If you are missing one of these ingredients, don't worry, any combination of the three, or even if you have only one, will do. If you'd like, you can add some healing herbs, such as Lavender or Chamomile, in there but you want to make sure to grind the herbs into a fine powder in your clean coffee grinder ahead of time. You can also store the powder that you make in a container with a cotton ball that has a few drops of essential oil on it to infuse the powder.

Non-Mineral Baby Oil

We've already discussed the problems with using mineral (petroleum byproducts) oils on our bodies so of course we don't want to use them on our babies either.

If you want a nice, non-mineral baby oil to soothe and soften your baby's skin after a bath it's as simple as getting some vegetable oil (such as olive oil or almond oil) and adding a little Vitamin E to it. This will nourish and soften your baby's skin as well as help to moisturize and heal it. Almond oil is very good to use because it absorbs easily into the skin and doesn't leave it feeling greasy.

Baby Bottom Balm

This balm has herbs in it that will soften and soothe baby's skin.

2 cups extra virgin olive oil (or almond oil)
1/3 cup Calendula
1/3 cup Rose Petals
1/3 cup Chamomile
6 capsules vitamin E (or ¼ cup vitamin E oil)
A few drops Lavender essential Oil
Enough beeswax to make salve the right consistency

This is made pretty much exactly like the previous baby balm. Combine the herbs and oil in a saucepan or slow cooker. You can use a double boiler also. Place on the lowest heat setting possible. You want to heat the oil enough to infuse the herbs but you don't want to fry them. Let the herbs infuse for about 3 hours but keep an eye on them to make sure the heat is not too high. When they are thoroughly infused remove them from the heat and allow the infusion to cool off. Once it's cool you can strain out the herbs. At this time you can add in the Vitamin E oil and the Lavender Essential Oil. Now, you'll want to put the oil back on a very slight heat, just enough to warm it up (you don't want to cook the essential oil out of it) and slowly add in the beeswax until it is completely melted. You can then pour the salve into your prepared containers and let it sit to solidify. If you've used too little beeswax you can warm it up again and add a little more. If you've found you've used too much beeswax then just make up a bit more oil, heat up the salve and add some of the new batch of oil to it. You may have to experiment with this a couple of times to get it precise.

* * *

Body After Pregnancy

Once the baby is born taking care of your body doesn't stop there. You're hormones will go back to some semblance of normal but your body has been through many changes.

When dealing with your complexion, remember that because of the hormonal differences after your pregnancy your skin may change. Just because you had oily or maybe dry skin before your pregnancy doesn't mean that will be the case afterward. Keep an eye on how your skin is reacting and adjust your skin care regimen accordingly.

If you have taken precautions during your pregnancy, such as eating right, exercising (if possible), using things like the Stretch Marks B-Gone Pregnant Belly Oil, you shouldn't have much problem getting your pre-pregnancy body back or even making it better.

If you have not had the chance to do those things there is still hope. By eating right, getting enough exercise and taking care of your skin you can tighten, soften and make your body healthier.

Find some exercises that you enjoy doing and that tighten up the certain areas of your body that you wish to focus on. Walking and swimming are two exercises that are not only good for you but can be very enjoyable also. If you can find a buddy to do these exercises with it will not only help you to remember to do them but it may also increase your enjoyment of them. Thirty minutes of exercise a day for around 3-5 days a week can do a lot of good for your body and really isn't that much time out of your day. Most people watch television or sit at their computers more than that. Exercise also increases endorphin production in the brain and can help to keep away postpartum depression.

Also make sure that you're getting enough water. It is recommended that you get at least 64 ounces of water a day. Now this may sound like a lot but when you break it down, it really isn't. I buy bottled water in bulk. I get thirty-two 16.9 ounce bottles of water in one package. I need to drink approximately 4 bottles of water a day to get my proper intake. I thought it would be difficult but I find myself drinking around 4-6 bottles a day. Now, I don't usually drink soda or fruit juices because of the sugar content. We all know soda isn't good for you and I prefer to eat whole fruit so that I get the full nourishment rather than just the juice mixed with water, sugar and preservatives.

There is a fruit juice that I do enjoy drinking when I choose to do so and that is Simply Orange, the high pulp version.

Because it has the pulp in it, I get some of the fiber that I would get if I ate an orange. Also, if you look at their ingredients all you'll find is 100% orange juice. They have other types of orange juices, lemonade, limeade, grapefruit and apple juices as well as a raspberry lemonade that we can't keep enough of in our home. Now, these are not organically grown but they do taste delicious and should be able to be found easily in your local grocery store.

* * *

Dealing with Menstruation

As we discussed in the previous chapter, many of us have come to see menstruation as something we have to "deal with". I think we need to be re-educated about our monthly cycles. In ancient days this time of the month was considered a sacred time when a woman was filled with power.

Your moon time, as it was often called, is a time of renewal. Your body is shedding tissue it no longer needs and this can be a time that works for you magickally as well. If you are harboring feelings of anger (after PMS who isn't?), resentment, or anything negative, this is a wonderful time to let those feelings go. Some women's cycles will even follow the moon's own cycles; ovulating around the full moon and getting blood flow at the waxing moon.

As tempting as not having a menstrual cycle might be to some it is not a good thing. If your body is not able to shed the lining it has created then that lining will begin to deteriorate inside you and can lead to things such as uterine cancer. By sloughing off those cells, it's similar to sloughing off the dead cells when you scrub your body or face. You can feel rejuvenated and renewed.

Using the more natural products that were discussed in the Maiden chapter may make you feel better about your cycle too. We need to take back the power that Mother Goddess has given us. These are our bodies and we have been given the power to bring forth life just as she did. Our cycles are not a curse but a reminder of our womanhood, our Goddess-ness. Throw off the shackles of patriarchal tyranny that we have been held down by. Woman is not the progenitor of sin. We are the creators of life. There is a story that says when one woman ate a fruit from a tree that gave her knowledge equal to that of a divine being and then brought that same fruit to the man that she loved she was punished for gaining said knowledge. She was punished by those who wished to hold her down and make her forget that knowledge and not be able to pass it on to her daughters and her daughters' daughters. Womanhood is not an affliction thrust upon us by a vengeful deity, as we have been led to believe. Womanhood is natural, beautiful, painful and empowering. We are mothers, daughters, sisters, grandmothers, friends and we should rejoice in the Goddess within us.

In the past (as well as still today) women were feared because of this power we hold. We have been taught to fear our own power and view it as something disgusting and dirty. I say NO MORE.

We hold the power. We hold the power of life, seduction, wrath and we have just as much right to wield those powers as anyone else. So, try to think about that the next time you get your cycle. Yes, we feel bloated and ugly, cranky and emotional but our menstrual cycle is part of the natural cycle of life. When you're hormones are in balance these complications are less likely to occur. If we eat healthy foods, stay hydrated and take care of our bodies things like

PMS or PMDD (Premenstrual Dysphoric Disorder) become virtually nonexistent.

If you find that you are having issues with PMS or PMDD try using some well known natural remedies to help solve these problems and get you back to living as the powerful and beautiful being that you are. Also, you may want to work on getting those hormones in balance so that you can prevent the symptoms from returning each month.

We can also have the power of knowing our cycles through natural family planning. This can be used if you want to have children or if not. You are in control. It is not 100% effective but nothing ever is. It will help for you to know your body better and may even help determine if there is something wrong.

* * *

Keeping your looks

Stress can do some really nasty things to our bodies. It affects our immune systems and can affect our skin as well. Our skin's ability to bounce back from things decreases as our bodies get older. This is an issue that I know some mothers are concerned over. There are some of us who enjoy our laugh lines and crow's feet because it reminds us of the good times we had in our lives but there are others who would prefer that these lines not be so prominent. There are even facial exercises that you can do to tone up your facial muscles as well as reduce wrinkles, laugh lines and the like.

At this point in your life you may think that you are too young to be bothered by these things but this information is good to have at any age.

Just like everything else, there are a ton of chemical laden products on the market to make your skin look and feel younger, etc. but these products can do more damage than good in the end.

We all know that one of the most important things you can do to keep healthy, young skin is to eat a good diet. This serves two purposes. It keeps you healthy and looking good but it also teaches your children to eat a healthy diet so that they can have long happy lives. I think that we can agree that children will live the way they learn and as parents we sometimes forget these things. You may not think your children are paying attention but they see things that we don't think about. So try to cultivate good habits from the start and you will be teaching your children valuable lessons that they can continue on in their adult lives.

Another thing that you want to do is to treat your skin right. Using natural facial scrubs, toners and moisturizers will do wonders for your skin, your health and possibly your outlook in general. Most of the things we find in the popular markets really are too harsh and some people can have adverse reactions to them.

Why not try some simple things you can make at home with everyday ingredients and see just how much better your skin, and your conscience, feels.

Exfoliating Facial/Body Scrub

This is a simple scrub that can be made quickly and is gentle enough to be used on the face as well as the body.

¼ Cup old fashioned rolled oats (ground fine)
¼ Cup powdered milk
1 Tablespoon salt
1 Tablespoon cornmeal

Mix all ingredients together and, when you shower or wash your face, take a small amount into the palm of your hand. Mix with a small amount of water and use to scrub your face or body.

After you scrub your face you are going to want to use some toner and then a moisturizer to get your skin's pH balance to where it should be.

Not all scrubs are created equal. This recipe is for one that can be used on both your face and your body but some body scrubs have ingredients that may be too rough to use on the sensitive skin of your face. For example, if your scrub contains coffee grounds you'll want to keep that away from your face.

Morning Oatmeal Facial Scrub

1 teaspoon Milk (whole milk for dry skin or skim milk for oily skin)
1 teaspoon rolled oats (ground fine in coffee grinder)
1 teaspoon almonds (ground fine in coffee grinder) or almond meal (optional)

Combine the ingredients, mix thoroughly and apply to face. You'll want to refrigerate this mixture if there is any left but probably shouldn't keep it more than a couple of days.

If you'd like to make a similar scrub that you can keep for longer you can use dry milk and reconstitute it with water. Just remember that most dry milk is made with nonfat milk and so it won't have the same properties as using whole milk.

Simple Skin Toner

1 teaspoon Apple Cider Vinegar
1 Cup water

Combine the two ingredients, mix thoroughly and apply with a spray bottle or a cotton ball. You'll want to refrigerate this mixture but probably shouldn't keep it more than a week.

Easy Honey & Egg Moisturizer

2 Tablespoon Honey
1 egg yolk

Mix the two ingredients together. They will form a paste that you want to apply to your face and neck. As with anything you put on your face, you want to avoid your eyes. Leave this on for about 15 minutes and then rinse it off.

Egg yolks contain Vitamin E and will do a good job of softening your skin. Honey is a humectant and will help to moisturize the skin.

If you follow good guidelines on keeping yourself and your skin healthy you will be less likely to "look your age". Starting early helps but if you are just now getting into it that doesn't mean that it's too late. It is never too late to start taking care of yourself.

* * *

Going Gray

Inevitably, it happens to all of us. For some it may be very early on in life and for others it may not happen until we are much older. There are many factors that will determine when your hair will actually begin to turn gray. Some of those factors can be the amount of stress you allow in your life, how healthy you keep your body and mind or how often you go outside.

Just as with wrinkles and laugh lines, some women are proud of their gray hair. Centuries ago, gray hair was often a sign of wisdom. Some I know have stated this must be because if you were able to live that long you must have been smart!

As usual, there are plenty of hair dyes out there that boast natural ingredients or vitamins in their product but if you look through their ingredients list there are probably quite a few ingredients that, not only do you not know what it is but, you can't pronounce them. Americans alone spend over a billion dollars a year on hair coloring. Most of these products contain hydrogen peroxide and ammonia, both of which can dry out and damage your hair. Even those companies who have "Natural Ingredients to help strengthen your hair" on the boxes still have dangerous chemicals in them that will damage it. The "natural" ingredients that they are claiming as such a big part of their advertising is often just as negligible as those from the other cosmetic and food companies.

Not only are we putting these damaging chemicals on our hair, on our skin, into the air we breathe but when we rinse our hair out we are washing those same chemicals down our drains. Out of sight, out of mind, right? Wrong! When we wash out these chemicals that we are warned not to breathe in or get on our skin (the instructions even tell you not to rub it into your scalp because it can be a major skin irritant) we are washing them into our drinking water and our water sources. Also, research has gone into whether or not these dyes contribute to certain types of cancer.

My maternal great grandmother (we called her Granny, a nickname that was started by my mother because she reminded her of the little old woman from The Beverly Hillbillies) was so against letting her hair go gray that she constantly dyed it. When she passed away, at the age of 95, it was the first time I had ever seen her with gray hair. The problem is that her hair became very thin. I remember watching her comb it out and wondering where the rest of it was.

If you are not one of those women who revels in your silvery colored locks or if you are just not ready to deal with having gray hair yet there are some things that you can do to help cover the gray that are much less harmful than what you can find on your local big store shelves.

Though these processes are not permanent they do provide more natural colors and are much safer to use.

Hair rinses are most commonly used with natural ingredients. In order to perform a hair rinse properly what you will want to do is to gather the juice or make an infusion, or tea, with the material you want to work with. You will want to combine these ingredients with water and use two large bowls in order to pour and catch the rinse. When you have your rinse ready, put your head over the bowl and pour the rinse, from one bowl, over your hair and into the other bowl below you. You'll then want to switch out the bowls and repeat the process. It is often recommended to repeat this process 15-20 times for the best results. Afterward, you will want to leave the rinse in your hair for about 15-20 minutes before rinsing with clear water. You may have to repeat this process over a couple of weeks to get the most out of it. There is no set period of time you'll need to continue this but keep an eye on your hair and you can continue the process until you get as close to the desired color as you want to be.

Natural rinses will fade with time so this is a process that you will need to do again once in a while. It is a good way to take time out and pamper yourself.

Hair Lightening Rinses

To lighten your hair you can do several things. Here are some rinses that can help to add blonde highlights to your hair.

Lemon Water Rinse

Juice of 2 lemons
1 quart water

Combine the strained lemon juice with the quart of water and follow the instructions on the previous page to rinse your hair.

Lemon Chamomile Rinse

½ cup Chamomile Flowers
1 quart water
1 cup lemon juice

Bring the quart of water to a boil and remove from heat. Add the Chamomile flowers to the water and let it steep for approximately thirty minutes. This can also be substituted with 3 cups of Chamomile Tea that you'll want to brew according to the instructions on the package. Let it sit and cool so that you won't burn yourself. Combine lemon juice with the chamomile tea, rinse your hair using the above instructions but when it comes time to let it sit you'll want to go outside for about an hour and sit in the sun. The sunlight will help to activate the lemon and chamomile to do their job. Afterward, rinse and condition your hair.

Both the Lemon Water Rinse and the Lemon Chamomile Rinse are best done in the summer time because, to get the most benefit, you will require help from the sun.

You can use plants other than chamomile, although it is the most popular. Pretty much any yellow flowered plant or herb will do. Some examples are Calendula (Pot Marigold), Turmeric and Mullein flowers.

Darkening The Hair

If you have dark hair and would like to enhance it or possibly would like to cover some of the gray sneaking up on you, sage is a great and effective herb to use. You can use it much the same as the Chamomile rinse.

Sage Darkening Hair Rinse

1 cup sage leaves

1 quart water

Bring the water to a boil and remove from heat. Add the sage to the water and let it steep for approximately thirty minutes. If you want a darker shade you will want to let it steep a bit longer. Let it sit and cool so that you won't burn yourself. Rinse your hair following the instructions on hair rinsing on page 117.

Some people also use black walnut hulls, coffee, tea, ground cloves or allspice to help enhance this same treatment.

Redheads

If you have red hair or want to add a red tint to your hair you can use things like hibiscus flowers, saffron, turmeric, calendula, carrot juice, beet juice or any other natural ingredient (or combination thereof) such as these that have a red hue to enhance your color. You may also use some of the same things, such as coffee or tea, which are recommended for brunettes. Remember to do a patch test first to make sure that you are getting as close to your desired color as possible.

Henna

Oftentimes it is not recommended to use Henna on gray or very light colored hair because it is very strong and, by itself, lends a brassy reddish orange color to the hair.

Mixed with other herbs Henna can lend an auburn color to the hair or carry with it the properties of the other herbs.

Before dying your hair you will want to perform a patch test to see what color the current recipe you have will bring out so that you can adjust it as needed. In order to do this you'll want to take a small patch of hair near the nape of the neck where it is less likely to be seen. Apply the dye there as you would normally. Wait the appropriate time and then check the hair to see if it is the color that you desire.

When mixing up a henna dye you will want to mix, into a bowl, one part powdered herb with two parts powdered henna. The bowl you use shouldn't be made of metal as this can cause discoloration due to the chemical reactions of the metal in the bowl with the natural chemicals in the herbs.

Add some boiling water to the mixture, enough to make a thick paste. If you'd like, you can also add a tablespoon or so of vinegar to the mixture. This will help to release the colors from the plants or herbs.

You'll want to wear rubber gloves when working with this mixture because it will stain your skin (as you may have seen with Henna tattoos, also known as Mehndi).

To start the dyeing process you'll want to have clean, dry hair. Apply the paste to your hair and massage it in. Run a comb through it to evenly distribute the paste. Take your hair and pile it on the top of your head. With a shower cap, plastic bag or even some plastic wrap from your kitchen, cover your hair and then wrap a towel around it to keep the heat in. The darker your natural hair is the longer you will have to leave this on, usually from half an hour to two hours.

When your time is up, rinse your hair thoroughly until the water runs clear. Afterward, let your hair air dry. If you find that you have accidentally stained your hands or the skin around your hairline you can scrub it with some lemon juice. The acids within the lemon juice should help get rid of the stains.

If this is a bit too much for you there are products, which you will usually find in health food shops, which use henna. The one that sticks in my mind most is Light Mountain. I have seen their product at the local health food co-operative in my home town. They use no ammonia and no peroxide and they even have a "Color the Gray" line of products.

* * *

Avoiding Empty Nest Syndrome

Throughout your life as a mother there are going to be things like soccer games, doctor's visits, skinned knees, first dates, first heartbreaks, good report cards, bad report cards, bullies, best friends one day and enemies the next, late nights, curfew breaks, sick babies (even if they **are** 15), bad music, shouts of "You don't understand!", finger paint on the curtains or crayon on the wall. Through it all, you will probably go through each and every up and down with your child, loving them the whole way even if some days you want to throttle them senseless.

As your children grow to the age where they will soon be leaving the nest you should remember some good advice that I received from a dear friend of mine. She had four children; two of them were teenagers and still living at home. She told me that one of the things she has had to keep in mind is to rediscover herself. In order to not get bogged down with empty nest syndrome she has to remember who she is other than just "Mom". She plans on going back to college as well as delving into some interests she has had for a long time but has been unable to pursue because her children came first.

You must remember that you are more than just a mom. You are probably also a daughter, sister, lover and friend. Motherhood is very important and a wonderful, stressful, beautiful thing that some women are able to experience in their life but it is not the end all be all to what their life is. Remember your own interests, hopes, goals and dreams. Even as a mother you can still reach for the stars, still feel beautiful and pursue your own interests.

As we move on through motherhood, some women look forward to the time when their monthly cycles will stop and they will enter Cronehood. Some women fear this part of their lives. In the next chapter we will discuss, in a more positive manner, the pros and cons of Cronehood and how to deal with some of the things that go with it.

Bewitching Beauty by Starr Morgayne

Crone

After Motherhood we begin to transition into the realm of the Crone. In modern culture we have been taught that "crones" are grumpy, disagreeable, malicious, and often useless, ugly old women. Though it is possible that the word "crone" comes from an old insult, crones are not the "old hags" that we usually see plastered all around during the month of October. Becoming a Crone is when you are welcomed into the sisterhood of old wise women. Cronehood usually begins at the onset of menopause. For some women, this is one of the hardest stages of life to go through. In a society that touts that the younger and thinner you can be the more beautiful you are it's no wonder that many older women have self esteem issues along with the young girls. Something else to be concerned about is the health issues that plague us as we get older. If you watch television often you will see many commercials about which pill to take to stave off Osteoporosis or some other such disease that comes with age.

As we age certain things in our bodies begin to slow down. Metabolism is one of those things and usually starts within your 30s. I believe that the reason our bodies begin to slow down at a progressive rate is that Cronehood is a time of reflection. It is our Creator's way of saying, "Slow down. Stop and smell the roses for a while."

This period of your life is a time to reflect on the years that have passed, what you have accomplished, watching your children and grandchildren grow. In previous centuries the elders of the tribes were considered the wisest of the people because they had lived so long and seen so many things. They were teachers and healers. There is no reason that this idea should just be thrown to the wind today. I have learned many things from my mother, grandmother and great grandmother. The things that we learn can be adapted to go with today's society but in everything there is wisdom.

* * *

Crone Goddesses

The Crone Goddesses represent the final of the three aspects of womanhood and, for some, the scariest part of the life cycle. The Crone Goddesses represent death, destruction and decay in order to be reborn. They are associated with the color black, the seasons Autumn and

Winter, the waning and/or new moon and are often rulers of the Underworld of their cultures.

Baba Yaga ~ Baba Yaga is a Slavic Goddess associated with Autumn and Death and Rebirth. She is a wild and untamed Crone. She lived deep in birch woods (the wise old woman of the forest) and possessed the Water of Life that she would sprinkle onto corpses for them to be reborn.

Cailleach ~ A Celtic Goddess of weather magic and seasonal rites, Cailleach was also known as the Bear Goddess. She governed over inner knowing and dreams. She is reborn each Samhain to bring about winter and each Spring turns into stone.

Elli ~ Elli is a Nordic Goddess of old age. It is said that she defeated the mighty Thor in a wrestling match showing that the strength of an older woman is still a powerful thing.

Hecate ~ Hecate is a Greek Goddess of the Crossroads. She is sometimes depicted with 3 heads which allows her to see more than most. She is a Goddess of wisdom though not conventionally.

Just like all of the other Goddesses we have spoken of here this is only a short list. There are innumerable lists of Goddesses for each aspect of womanhood. Find ones that speak to you and whatever path you are on.

* * *

Skin Care

Your skin probably needs a bit more TLC at this point in your life. There are many things that you can do to help with that. If you are lucky and have had previous knowledge you may have been following some of the steps to keep your skin healthy long before now. If not, don't despair. It's never too late to start a good regimen and make your skin as healthy as possible at any age.

As we mature our skin begins to lose some of its moisture. It becomes drier, more wrinkled, loses its elasticity, tends to heal more slowly and we may develop spots or growths. Make sure to stay hydrated in order to combat some of this from the inside out.

Dry Skin

When you have trouble with dry skin you want to make sure to use a good humectant. A humectant will help to hold moisture within the skin tissue. A good moisturizer will do wonders for you skin.

When you bathe make sure not to use hot water. Hot water dries out the skin as do commercial soaps. Try to use warm water and a mild soap when you bathe.

Avocados are really great for dry mature skin or even oily skin. What you'll want to do is pick a nice ripe avocado, scoop out the flesh, mash it up and apply it on your skin. It makes a really great facial mask. Leave it on for ten or fifteen minutes and sit back and relax. When you're ready you'll want to soften it with some warm water and gently wipe it off with a warm washcloth and pat your skin dry. If your skin is extremely dry you might want to mix some olive oil in with the avocado.

Dry Skin Mask

1 Tbsp rolled oats
1 tsp honey
¼ banana

This is a great quick and easy mask. The first step is to take the rolled oats and grind them into a fine powder in your coffee grinder. Then peel and cut up your banana and drop it into a blender. Pour the honey and oatmeal powder in and blend to a smooth consistency. Apply all over the face and let sit for 20 minutes. Gently rinse with warm water.

These three ingredients make an excellent mask for dry skin for several reasons and if you make too much to use in one sitting you can always eat what is left!

Bananas are good sources of many different vitamins such as A, B, C and E as well as minerals which are very good for not only the inside of your body but the outside too. They help to soften and moisturize the skin therefore helping to combat early aging and wrinkles.

Honey is a humectant that draws moisture from the air and into the skin. It also has antibacterial properties which help to combat blemishes, pimples, whiteheads, etc.

Oats have been used for centuries for skin care and healing. They soothe, moisturize and soften the skin.

If you like you can even throw a little yogurt into this recipe for its moisturizing properties.

Wrinkles

As we age our skin loses its elasticity and begins to look loose, become thinner and loses fat so the plump smooth look we use to have fades. Gravity pulls on the skin causing it to sag. Overexposure to the sun, stress, overly processed foods, overindulgence in alcohol and smoking can also cause damage to the skin. Some of it is even hereditary.

You can help to prevent wrinkles in several ways. You can protect yourself from the sun by using sunscreens and/or limiting your exposure. Alpha hydroxy acids have been shown to reduce and sometimes reverse some of the effects of the sun on skin.

In order to help our bodies produce more collagen and plump up those wrinkles we can increase our intake of Vitamin C which is a necessary ingredient for our body to make collagen. Adding more fresh fruits and vegetables to your diet will increase the amount of antioxidants you are getting.

Here is a great wrinkle treatment using some items easily found in the local grocery aisles.

Wrinkle Treatment

A few carrots

Some slices of cucumber

Throw the carrots and cucumber into a food processor and grind them into mush. Apply them to your skin and leave on for about 20 minutes. Gently wash them off when the time is up.

Some other foods you can use in this manner are grapes, papaya, oatmeal, olive oil and purslane.

Liver Spots

"Liver spots" or "age spots" as they are sometimes called, actually have nothing to do with the liver. They normally appear on the face, hands, feet and back and are generally harmless. They are caused by the sun. If you want to try to fade them a bit don't run out to the local store and by a "fade cream". Just mix up some lemon juice and yogurt and apply it to the skin. Leave on for about 20 minutes and gently rinse off. If you do this over several days you may see the spot begin to fade. It is not likely to get rid of the spot completely though it can make you feel better just to lighten it a bit.

Remember that as we age our skin can become more sensitive to fabrics, chemicals, weather and many things in our environment. Take care of your skin and protect it.

* * *

Varicose Veins

Though not a skin care issue, I felt that this topic was one that should at least get a mention in this chapter. They don't look very attractive and can be lessened by doing some very simple things.

Varicose veins are found in the legs and tend to bulge out and be blue in color. They are very common and are caused by the blood in the veins returning to the heart, against gravity, flowing back into the veins through a faulty valve.

A couple of the best ways to combat Varicose Veins, and the achiness associated with them, is to try to keep from standing for long periods of time and to keep your feet elevated when you are lying down or sitting.

* * *

Menopause

As stated earlier, menopause is usually considered the beginning of Cronehood. Menopause is literally the cessation of menstruation. It is the time when women's bodies begin to produce less of the hormones estrogen and progesterone and she is no longer able to become pregnant. The process of Menopause, unlike Menarche, can take several years. It usually starts between the ages of 42 and 56 but can happen much earlier or later. In modern times menopause can be caused by surgery or other factors at a much earlier age than natural menopause. This is why menopause is, now, not the only consideration for Cronehood. The timing of when a woman becomes a Crone has to do with her readiness as well as her age.

The Croning Ritual

The Croning Ritual is a ritual in which you celebrate the knowledge and wisdom gained throughout your years of life. Your Croning Ritual may include anyone you chose; other crones, only women or women, men and children. This can be a time of chanting, drumming, taking on a "Crone Name", solitary reflection, commitment making, or anything you want it to be.

In Dorothy Morrison's book In Praise of the Crone there is a Croning Ritual that can be done alone. There are also options for women who would like to celebrate with friends.

There are many books out there with ideas for Croning Rituals or any other milestone of life rituals. My advice to you is this: You're a Crone! You have enough life experience that you can do whatever feels right to you and you know what? That's what's right! Celebrate your femininity, your wisdom, your life. Celebrate you because you deserve it!

* * *

Bewitching Beauty by Starr Morgayne

Afterword

This book is all about celebrating your own femininity and recognizing that the Goddess lives inside all of us no matter what stage of life we are in. We need to learn to live, love and laugh like the Goddesses we are. Celebrate who you are. Push to be the best you can be at whatever it is you choose to do. Perfection may be a goal we never reach but it can still be a goal that we strive for every day. Never forget that you are a unique and beautiful creature.

It is also about using things found in our natural environment to keep ourselves looking beautiful, connecting with our Mother Earth, and helping to live a more "green" lifestyle.

By doing all of these things we make our world a better place not only for ourselves but for our children, loved ones and all of the people around us. We can lead by example.

Bewitching Beauty by Starr Morgayne

Glossary of Terms

Analgesic – An analgesic reduces pain

Anti-inflammatory – An anti-inflammatory decreases inflammation.

Antibacterial – An antibacterial destroys or inhibits the growth of bacteria.

Antimicrobial – An antimicrobial destroys or inhibits the growth of micro-organisms

Antioxidant – An antioxidant is a substance that reduces the damage that oxygen does to the tissue, usually caused by free radicals which are chemicals that attack the molecules in your skin.

Antiseptic – Antiseptics help to prevent infection and to get rid of disease causing organisms.

Antiviral – Something that is antiviral kills or prevents a virus from multiplying.

Astringent – An astringent tightens soft tissue in order to slow the flow of secretions.

Decoction – A decoction is a type of tea made by boiling roots, barks, seeds, stems, berries or heartier parts of plants

Demulcent – A demulcent is soothing. Demulcents are usually used to soothe and soften inflamed skin.

Diaphoretic – A diaphoretic has the power to increase perspiration (sweating).

Emollient – An emollient softens and moisturizes the skin. It is usually found in the form of a lotion or thick liquid.

Emulsifier – An emulsifier allows ingredients that do not normally mix well to blend together. Example: oil and water.

Emulsion – A mixture of two (usually) liquids that don't normally mix. Example: oil and water.

Exfoliant – An exfoliant is an abrasive used to scrub the skin in order to remove dead skin cells and increase circulation.

Humectant – A humectant holds water or moisture (in this case it is something that will hold moisture to the skin)

Inflammation – The symptoms of inflammation are usually pain, swelling, redness and heat.

Infusion – In the case of this book an infusion is what you get when you use a liquid to pull the needed constituents out of plant matter and into the liquid. Example: tea

Maceration – Technically, maceration is the preparation of an extract by soaking the containing material in an organic solvent. This would include infusions, decoctions, tinctures etc. but in herbal terms it has come to mean, a cold infusion of herbs in water, oil or vinegar.

Poultice – A poultice is usually a warm, wet mass that is applied externally. It is most often on or in between cloth and used for inflamed areas of the body.

Salve – Merriam-Webster's Online Dictionary defines a salve as "an unctuous adhesive substance for application to wounds or sores." My definition of a salve is a mixture of plant matter infused in oil and combined with either beeswax or hydrogenated vegetable oil.

Steeping – Steeping is the process used to make an infusion. You would cover your plant matter with liquid and let it steep by letting it sit for however long is needed.

Tincture – A tincture is what you get when you infuse alcohol with plant matter.

Tools

Here is information on some of the tools that you might like to have when you are making your own skin care products. You will want to make sure that you have separate items for skin care product making than you use for cooking because some of the ingredients you use may become absorbed by the tools (most often wood or plastic) and won't bode well for your cooking. If you are using essential oils remember that they can melt plastic.

Coffee Grinder ~ One of my favorite and most used tools is my coffee grinder. I have one for my coffee (which I indulge in once in a great while) and a completely separate one for making skin care products. It is good for when I'm making baby powders, deodorant powders, grinding oatmeal to make it colloidal and so many other uses.

Wooden Spoons ~ Wooden spoons are good for stirring your mixtures because they won't impart some of the impurities that using metal or plastic will. However, they can soak up smells, essential oils and other constituents of whatever it is you are stirring.

Bowls ~ You'll need bowls to mix your ingredients. For some things you can use plastic bowls but for others you may want to use glass or ceramic.

Blender ~ A blender is good to have for making emulsions for lotions or creams. I have one blender for edible items and another (made of glass) for making my skin care products.

Cheesecloth ~ You can use this to make bath bags or tea bags. You just gather the herbs in the cloth and pull it up around them. You then tie it off with a string. Cheesecloth can also be used for straining oils or other liquids through.

Coffee filters ~ Used for straining, similar to cheesecloth.

Double Boiler ~ You can either buy a double boiler or just combine two pots. The pot on the bottom has water in it and the pot inside is where you put whatever it is you need to heat. A double boiler is used to keep sensitive ingredients from getting too hot and burning.

Strainers or colanders ~ You can add cheesecloth or coffee filters within the strainer to help strain the herb bits out of your oils.

Measuring cups and spoons ~ Liquid measuring cups can make certain ingredients easier to pour and if you have the glass ones you don't have to worry about them soaking up essential oils.

Funnels ~ Funnels make filling bottles so much easier and a lot less messy. You will want to have several different sizes.

Mortar & Pestle ~ Every Kitchen Witch should have a mortar and pestle. It is good to use to grind up those things that you just can't get ground properly in a food processor or coffee grinder (and it looks really witchy).

Pans ~ You can go with ceramic pans but you don't necessarily have to. Just remember that some metals may react adversely to some of the ingredients.

Bath Tea Bags ~ You don't necessarily have to have these but I love them. They're essentially large tea bags with drawstring closures. They're great for tossing in some herbs, colloidal oats and possibly some milk powder. You can even use them to scrub yourself with or just hang them from your faucet for the water to flow through into the bath (after you've closed them and tied a knot in the drawstring at the opening of the bag and the end of the string). They're easily found at your local superstore or craft store. You can also sometimes substitute cheesecloth or even a wash cloth that is tied up around whatever ingredients you are using.

French Press ~ This is a somewhat fancy and completely optional item to have on hand. I like to use mine for straining oils and teas because I can squeeze out more of the infusion than I could with cheesecloth. The cheesecloth tends to soak up some of the infusion and can let small particles through.

Ingredients

As stated before, many of the recipes used within this book contain common ingredients found in your local grocery store, pharmacy and/or health food store.

Here you will find a list of these products and what they are commonly used for as well as the magickal uses for some.

Almond ~ Almond meal is made from ground almonds. It is often used as an exfoliant and emollient in many facial scrubs. It is high in nutrients and fats that are good for the skin. Some of the Goddesses associated with almonds are Artemis, Cybele and Hecate.

Almond Oil, Sweet ~ Sweet Almond Oil (sometimes just called Almond Oil) is absorbed readily into the skin and makes a wonderful massage and carrier oil that is good for all skin types. It conditions, heals, revitalizes, smoothes and softens skin as well as being an emollient. One drawback is that it has a short shelf life.

Aloe Vera ~ Many of you are familiar with the Aloe Vera plant, its burn healing properties and its ability to help repair damaged tissue. Aloe draws and holds oxygen to the skin which aids in the healing process. The gel from the leaf can be used but you can also find Aloe Vera juice in many places. It is soothing, softening, astringent and rejuvenating. It helps to draw out infections and heals skin irritations. It can also help to combat wrinkles. Aloe is closely associated with the moon and lunar magick.

Apple Cider Vinegar ~ Apple Cider Vinegar is soothing and antiseptic. This valuable product helps to restore your skin's natural pH balance, relieve itchiness and is slightly astringent for those with normal to oily skin. It has been used for many years to help those afflicted with sunburn. One of my teachers advised me to take a shot of Apple Cider Vinegar a day to stay healthy. I couldn't manage it but some people can. You want to make sure to get a good, organic apple cider vinegar that still has the "mother" in it. This is the key component. You can either shoot it straight or dilute it in a glass of water.

Apples ~ Apples contain a compound known as malic acid which is an exfoliating enzyme. They are slightly astringent. Because of this, they are good at helping shed dead skin cells and bacteria. It also helps protect from infection by restoring your skin's natural acidity. Apples are associated with the Goddesses Venus, Athena, Hera and Aphrodite. They are often used in love and beauty spells.

Apricot ~ Apricots have moisturizing, revitalizing and nourishing properties and are good for oily skin. Used in love spells.

Arrowroot ~ The root of this plant is often used in powder form. It can be used in place of baby powder for a more natural alternative. Arrowroot can be used for spells of love, exorcism or to help with psychic powers.

Ascorbic Acid ~ Ascorbic Acid is Vitamin C. It can be used as a preservative in cosmetics and to adjust the skin's Ph balance.

Avocado ~ Avocado has nourishing and conditioning properties for both the skin and hair. The oil is used as an emollient. It is rich in proteins, minerals and vitamins and readily penetrates the skin. It is excellent for cracked or mature skin and heals, revitalizes and regenerates cells. It is an excellent oil for face and massage oils. Avocado can be used magickally for beauty, love and lust.

Baking Soda ~ Also known as Sodium Bicarbonate, baking soda has many properties. It softens water, deodorizes, and draws oils and impurities from the skin. It also is soothing, effervescent and stimulating. It can be used in bath powders or as a deodorant and tooth whitener. You can also use it to make your hair clean and shiny by mixing it with water to remove the nasty residues left behind from hairstyling products. Baking soda has so many uses that I couldn't possibly name them all here but check into it. You may be surprised.

Bananas ~ Bananas are moisturizing and nourishing to the skin. They are extremely gentle and are an emollient for both normal and dry skin. Bananas can be used magickally for fertility and prosperity.

Basil ~ Basil is often used to promote hair growth. It can be used in spells or rituals for love, wealth, purification and protection. It has been linked to the deity Vishnu.

Beeswax ~ Beeswax is commonly used as a thickener and an emulsifier for lotions, salves, etc. It helps to seal moisture within the skin but will still allow the skin to "breathe" unlike petroleum based products. It also has germ killing properties.

Beets ~ Beet juice is often used in hair washes to enhance red hair. Magickally, beets are associated with love.

Bentonite Clay ~ Bentonite is clay made from volcanic ash and is often used to make face masks.

Benzoin Gum ~ A preservative often used in cosmetics also known as Styrax. Magickally, benzoin is associated with prosperity and purification.

Black Walnut ~ Black Walnut, specifically the hull, is often used for its antifungal properties as well as its astringency. It was used in spells for protection, mental powers, health, infertility and wishes.

Borax ~ Borax is an emulsifier and also gently cleans without drying out your skin. The chemical name for borax is sodium borate or sodium tetraborate.

Burdock ~ Burdock is filled with nutrients. The leaves and root both have nutritional as well as medicinal properties. It has been known as a liver cleanser, diuretic and blood purifier. It has been known to act as a hypoglycemic (lowers blood sugar). It is also reported to increase hair growth, strength and sheen when used as a hair rinse. Magickal properties of Burdock are protection and healing.

Buttermilk ~ Buttermilk is used to exfoliate and soften the skin.

Calendula ~ Calendula (Calendula officinalis) is also known as Pot Marigold. It is very useful as a natural beauty tonic. It is anti-inflammatory, antiseptic, antifungal, antibacterial, cleansing, softening, smoothing as well as regenerative. It accelerates healing and can be used as a colorant. It is one of my favorite plants to use when making my own skin care products because it helps to tone and refresh the skin. It is useful in helping to prevent wrinkles and healing acne. Magickally, calendula is associated with protection, prophetic dreams, psychic powers and legal matters.

Carrots ~ Carrots have antiseptic, anti-aging, cleansing, moisturizing and nourishing properties. They are rich in vitamins A, B, C and beta-carotene. Carrot oil is used to help reduce scarring. Magickally, it is associated with fertility and lust.

Cashew ~ As with any nut, these can be ground into a fine powder and, added to other ingredients, make a nice exfoliant. Cashews are magickally associated with money.

Chamomile ~ Chamomile tea is a great anti-inflammatory for pimples/zits/acne and is good for helping you relax and sleep. It is mildly astringent, diaphoretic, restorative and healing. The flowering tops were often used for money, love and purification rituals and spells. It is also said to induce sleep when burned.

Cinnamon ~ Cinnamon is antiseptic, astringent and stimulating. The powder can be used as an exfoliant but be careful because it can also be very irritating. Magickally, cinnamon is associated with healing, psychic powers, success, power, lust, protection, exorcism, money, love and spirituality.

Clove ~ Cloves are antiseptic and their smell, usually brought out by using the essential oil, is used to calm and relieve stress. Magickally cloves are used for many things. They can be used in love, lust and attraction spells, protection, exorcism, money, driving away negativity and hostility and stopping gossip. Cloves can be carried to comfort you if you're in mourning or to stimulate the memory. The oil is wonderful for toothaches as well.

Cocoa Butter ~ Who doesn't love cocoa butter? I use it all the time to make many lotions. It has a wonderful smell and moisturizes and softens the skin. It is a humectant, as well as emollient, which makes it great for mature or cracked skin but use sparingly on oily skin. Also, because it is a heavy saturated fat, it should not be used on the face.

Coffee ~ Finely ground coffee grounds can be used, not only for their scent, but also as an exfoliant. It has recently been reported that using coffee in a body scrub helps to rid you of cellulite by increasing circulation and breaking up clusters of fat. It can even help to eliminate varicose veins by tightening and shrinking blood vessels.

Comfrey ~ Comfrey is used to soothe and lubricate dry skin. It is also helpful in cell regeneration. The leaf can be used as a compress for swelling and bruising. Comfrey is often used in sachets or spells for safe travel. You can put it in your luggage to help prevent it from being stolen. It often brings luck or money to the person carrying it.

Cornmeal ~ Cornmeal can be used as an exfoliating ingredient in body scrubs. Magickally it is used for protection, luck, and divination.

Cornstarch ~ Cornstarch is sometimes referred to as "corn flour". It is a "starchy" white powder that comes from corn and is very soothing to the skin. It is used as a thickening agent and can also be used as baby or body powder instead of talc. If you have an allergy to corn it is probably a good idea to do a patch test with this first as it may cause an allergic reaction.

Cucumber ~ Cucumbers are soothing, cleansing and toning. You'll want to leave the skin on the cucumber when you use it because it contains most of the vitamins and minerals. Cucumbers can help to make your skin less susceptible to acne by breaking down the bacteria with the

Vitamin C it contains. Cucumbers also keep skin healthy and help to maintain elasticity because of the potassium, sulfur and silicon contained in it. Cucumbers are associated with moon magick, chastity, healing and fertility.

Diatomaceous Earth ~ Diatomaceous Earth has so many uses. For skin care you can use it as a base for face masks but you can also sprinkle it on your garden for an earth friendly way to keep vegetable eating bugs away and you can sprinkle a little in your pets' food to take care of intestinal parasites. Make sure to get this from your health food store and do not use the Diatomaceous Earth you find near pool cleaning supplies.

Eggs ~ Eggs are very valuable, not only in our diet but also in our beauty regimen. They are nourishing, conditioning and astringent. They are useful in face masks, shampoos and hair conditioners. Make sure not to use them with hot ingredients though or you will cook them. Egg yolks contain Vitamin A, Vitamin B5, sulfur and lecithin which is an emollient. The Albumin (or egg white) has soothing and tightening properties for the skin.

Epsom Salt ~ Epsom salts are also known as magnesium sulfate and have been used for years to put into foot baths to soothe aching feet or in just your regular bath to pull impurities from the body. They can even be used to help constipation (please read the directions on the bag/box before trying this or consult your health care practitioner) or as a fertilizer. They are mildly astringent and help increase circulation.

Eucalyptus ~ Eucalyptus can be used in so many healing ways. You can make a salve with it to rub onto your chest as you sleep to make breathing easier and break up congestion or you can combine it with clove and peppermint for a sinus relieving bath. Magickally it is associated with healing and protection.

Fennel ~ Fennel has restorative, cleansing, detoxifying and antiseptic properties. It helps maintain the elasticity of the skin because of an estrogen-like substance it contains. All parts of the plant can be used. This herb has been used to ward off evil and negativity as well as protection, healing and purification.

Garlic ~ Because of garlic's healthful properties, in old days it was hung in rooms in order to ward off disease. This is why its magickal properties are protection and healing. It can also be used for anti-theft spells, banishing, lust and exorcism.

Glycerin ~ Glycerin is often used as a skin protectant. You should be able to find it in your local pharmacy. Glycerin attracts moisture and holds it which makes it a humectant.

Grape ~ Grape juice contains many Alpha Hydroxy Acids as well as Vitamin C. Deities: Dionysus, Bacchus, Hathor. Magickal Associations: Fertility, Garden Magic, Mental Powers, Money

Green Tea ~ Green Tea has become popular in recent years because of its antioxidant properties. It is also popular belief that Green Tea has anti-aging properties. It can be used as a face rinse to tighten the pores.

Honey ~ Honey has many wonderful properties. It is antibacterial, emollient, moisturizing, nourishing, soothing and cleansing. It also promotes healing. In ancient times it was thought to be "the food of the Gods" and what made them immortal. The Romans believed that using honey on your skin made you more attractive especially when mixed with olive oil. Honey is one of the best known humectants and is high in potassium, therefore making it difficult for bacteria to survive in it. Also, if you want to sweeten your medicinal teas you should use honey instead of sugar. Sugar has components in it that break down the medicinal properties in the teas and make them no longer work. Honey, on the other hand, does not and is healthier for you than sugar.

Jasmine ~ Jasmine has been used magickally for love, money, prophetic dreams. It is said that you can use a drop of Jasmine essential oil in almond oil, massage it into the skin and this will help overcome frigidity. Deity: Vishnu

Jojoba Oil ~ Jojoba is very similar to the natural oil that is secreted by your skin daily. Because of this, it is easily absorbed by the skin. Jojoba is a natural moisturizer and helps with renewal of skin cells. It also has antioxidant properties and is great for treating acne and problems such as eczema, psoriasis and dry skin.

Lavender ~ Lavender is one of my most favorite herbs. It is one of the few essential oils you can use neat (by itself, without diluting in a carrier oil) on the skin. It has so many wonderful properties. It is anti-inflammatory, antibacterial, antiseptic, balancing, relaxing, soothing. It helps both dry and oily skin by helping to normalize secretions from the sebaceous glands. It also stimulates growth of new cells. It can be used to repel insects as well as to calm yourself and reduce stress. Lavender can help with sinus issues and headaches. If you are having trouble with either one take a couple drops of Lavender oil and put them on your temples and rub under your eyes. This should help clear up the issue in no time. It is used magickally for purification, chastity (by sprinkling lavender water on the head), sleep (burning for relaxation), maintain a peaceful and harmonious home, and bringing strength and courage.

Lemon ~ Lemon has antiseptic, rejuvenating, stimulating, astringent and mild bleaching properties. It also helps to restore the natural acid balance of the skin because it contains Citric Acid which is an AHA or alpha hydroxy acid and BHA or beta hydroxy acid. Citric Acid kills bacteria on the skin. Be careful though because citrus oils may irritate sensitive skins and cause photosensitivity.

Also, don't use on sore or irritated skin. The scent of lemon is used in aromatherapy for its uplifting and refreshing effects. Lemon peel is magickally associated with longevity, purification, love and friendship.

Lemon Balm ~ Also known as Bee Balm or Melissa (it's Latin name is Melissa Officinalis), Lemon Balm is part of the mint family and is said to be antiviral. Studies have shown that putting a salve of Lemon Balm on herpes sores can make a huge difference in healing them and possibly help to keep them from returning. Lemon Balm is used magickally in success and healing spells as well as to find love and friendship.

Lemongrass ~ Lemongrass is said to be antifungal, analgesic, astringent and can increase circulation. Magickally, Lemongrass is used to increase lust and psychic powers as well as to repel snakes.

Loofah ~ You see Loofah sponges on store shelves all over but did you know that they're not really sponges at all? They're actually gourds that you can grow yourself. When dried, you can chop them into small bits and put them in your scrubs to make a good Exfoliant or you can slice them or use them whole to scrub your body. Make sure not to use it on your face though, it's too harsh.

Marshmallow ~ This is not the fluffy white things you roast over camp fires but it is a very useful root. I have used it in baby baths because it helps to soothe the skin and soften it. The marshmallows we know today came about because Marshmallow root used to be cut into squares, boiled (which caused them to puff up) and then rolled in powdered sugar so they didn't stick together in the container they were stored in. They were given to help with stomach troubles.

Mayonnaise ~ Mayonnaise can be used as a skin and/or hair conditioner. The ingredients in mayonnaise (eggs, oil, lemon juice and vinegar) are all good for the skin and hair. Make sure to check out their individual properties also.

Milk ~ Milk has been used in ancient times, and even now, in baths to soothe irritated skin as well as soften it. Milk contains an alpha hydroxyl acid known as lactose which gently sloughs off dead skin cells. Using milk to moisturize and soften the skin was originally made popular by

Cleopatra in Egypt. Milk is associated with fertility (of body, life, etc.)

Mint ~ Members of the mint family tend to be naturally astringent as well as refreshing. They are good to use to boost your mood or wake you up.

Nettle ~ Nettle leaf is best used fresh. It is full of nutrients and is often used to help with women's hormonal imbalances. Nettle is used magickally for exorcism (usually burned during ceremonies), protection (by sprinkling around the room), healing and lust.

Oats ~ For centuries, oats have been used for their skin-soothing properties. They are exceptionally healing, soothing and exfoliating. You can get (or make) 3 different types of ground oatmeal; fine, medium and coarse. If you're using it for a facial scrub you'll want to use the fine (or colloidal) so as not to damage the delicate skin of the face. You can use the medium or coarsely ground for body scrubs. You can grind your own oatmeal (using rolled oats from the grocery) with a common coffee grinder. It is especially good for sensitive skin. Oats are magickally associated with money.

Olive Oil ~ Olive Oil is often used as an emollient and it attracts moisture to the skin. It has a long shelf life and blends well with other oils. I like to use Extra Virgin Olive Oil. You can often store Olive Oil, without refrigeration, for up to a year. It is especially good for dry skin and makes an excellent conditioner for nails and hair.

Onion ~ Onions are anti-bacterial and pull impurities from the skin. For example, if you are stung by a bee or bitten by an insect you can cut an onion in half and hold it on the wound for about 10 minutes. You'll want to do this as soon as possible to get as much of the toxins out as you can. Onions are magickally associated with protection.

Orange ~ The scent of an orange is very uplifting and refreshing. To get the scent you can use essential oil or orange zest (the peel). Orange peel is used magickally for love, divination, luck and money.

Papaya ~ Papaya pulp contains an enzyme called "papain" that is protein-digesting, which helps dissolve the dead outer layer of skin, exfoliating, rejuvenating and healing the skin. It may irritate sensitive skin so make sure that before using it you do a patch test. Also restores the skin's natural pH level. Magickally associated with moon magick, love and protection.

Parsley ~ Parsley, like the members of the mint family, is naturally astringent. It can also be soothing and healing for those who suffer with bad cases of acne, eczema and psoriasis. Ever wonder why restaurants put Parsley as a garnish on the plates? It's not just there to look pretty. Parsley freshens your breath after a meal. Parsley also makes a good rinse for all hair types. It is often used in love magick, protection and purification spells. Deity: Persephone

Peach ~ Peaches have chemicals within them, such as alpha-hydroxy acids, that help to slough off old skin cells and reveal newer fresher skin. They can help to get rid of lines and wrinkles in your face. The pulp can be moisturizing and lightly toning for the skin. Magickal properties include love, exorcism, longevity, fertility, and wishes

Peanut ~ As with any nut, these can be ground into a fine powder and, added to other ingredients, make a nice exfoliant.

Pear ~ Pears can be used to exfoliate the skin. Magickal aspects include love and lust.

Peppermint ~ Peppermint is invigorating, cooling, anti-inflammatory, analgesic and mildly antiseptic. It's good for helping to get rid of aches and pains as well as controlling bacteria on the skin. Magickal uses of Peppermint are many and varied. It is a great mental stimulant and therefore is often used to enhance psychic powers and awareness. It is used in cleansing incenses as well as charms to help heal the sick. The essential oil has been used in spells to bring about positive changes.

Pineapple ~ Pineapple has cleansing, rejuvenating and exfoliating properties. It revitalizes the skin and has many enzymes, vitamins and minerals. It is good for oil and acne prone complexions because it dissolves oil, bacteria and dirt. Magickal aspects include luck, chastity and money.

Potato ~ Potatoes are soothing, softening and anti-inflammatory. They are a major source of B vitamins which, when eaten, help to deal with stress and, when applied to the skin, help reduce oiliness and blackhead formation on the face. The peels can be boiled to make a hair rinse that is conditioning as well as darkening. Potatoes are often used as poppets or voodoo dolls. Other magickal associations are healing, protection and grounding.

Pumpkin ~ Pumpkin is a powerful antioxidant and helps to accelerate exfoliation. Pumpkin seeds can be a great snack and are said to increase fertility.

Raspberry ~ Raspberry leaf tea has been used to help many women's issues. It is said to help with hormone imbalances, menstrual cramps as well as childbirth. You can find it often combined with Nettle. Raspberry brambles have been hung at the entrances to homes in order to prevent unwanted spirits from entering. As a food, raspberries have been thought to induce love.

Rose ~ Roses have long been associated with love and beauty. The essence of roses has been used for centuries for such things as relieving depression and grief, attracting love and passion, as an aphrodisiac as well as symbolizing beauty. Some say that rose oil is one of the first essential oils documented for use. You can use them to make rose water which can be a wonderful toner to the skin, especially when combined with glycerin. If you decide that you would like to try to make your own rose water make sure to use organically grown roses so that you won't be adding pesticides and other harsh chemicals to your skin. Magickally they are associated with love, psychic powers, healing, divination, luck and protection. They are also associated with the Zodiac signs Taurus, Cancer, Libra and Sagittarius. It should also come as no surprise that roses are associated with the planet Venus. Deities: Hathor, Hulda, Eros, Cupid, Demeter, Isis, Adonis, Harpocrates, Aurora

Rosemary ~ Rosemary has astringent, antiseptic, detoxifying and stimulating properties. It helps to rid the skin of impurities by opening the pores and helps to prevent wrinkles. It is very helpful for oily skin and is a strong antioxidant. Rosemary is known to improve circulation as well as promoting hair growth and conditioning hair. I like to put a couple of drops of rosemary essential oil in my shampoo. Rosemary has many magickal properties such as love, protection, banishment, lust, increasing mental powers, healing, and attracting elves.

Sage ~ Sage has been used to darken and tone hair as well as being a hair growth stimulant. It also has antibacterial properties. Magickally, sage has a myriad of uses. It is used to consecrate sacred areas and to remove impurities from the air, banish evil and provide protection by burning in smudge sticks. Other magickal properties of sage are wisdom, longevity, immortality and prosperity.

Salt ~ Salt is astringent and antiseptic. It can be used as an exfoliant for dead skin cells but don't use it on your face because it can be too drying. All salts have detoxifying and muscle-relaxing properties but make sure that you do not use salt on your skin after shaving. Ouch! Table salt is chemically known as sodium chloride. Sea Salt softens and re-adds minerals to the skin.

Sour Cream ~ Sour Cream is used to exfoliate and soften the skin.

Strawberry ~ Strawberries can be used to whiten teeth by mashing them with a fork and then brushing your teeth with the pulp. They can also help to stimulate the skin by giving it Vitamin C which helps to reduce swelling, redness, stress and gives your skin a nice glow. They also contain sulfur, which has cleansing and anti-inflammatory properties that help to remove impurities from the skin's surface and reduce redness and swelling. Strawberries gently exfoliate the skin through natural fruit acids and enzymes. Strawberries are magickally associated with love, luck and the Goddess Freya.

Sunflower Seed Meal ~ Sunflowers contain oils that are good for the skin. Make sure to use raw sunflower seeds when you grind them into meal. Sunflower seeds are used magickally for fertility, health and wisdom.

Tea Tree – Tea Tree oil is also known as melaleuca oil and is native to Australia. It is antiseptic, antifungal, antibacterial and antiviral. It is easily absorbed by the skin and, along with lavender, can be used neat (by itself, without diluting in a carrier oil). I use a few drops of it in shampoo to help with dandruff. Tea Tree has been used as an antiseptic, fungicide and germicide.

Tomato ~ Tomato juice contains vitamins C, E and B3 as well as Lycopene. Lycopene protects the skin from sun damage and also helps to prevent wrinkles. Magickally tomatoes represent prosperity, protection and love. The use of tomato for skin care is ideal because of its cooling and astringent properties. The Vitamin C contained in it makes it helpful for acne and brightening dull skin. Its naturally acidic properties help it balance the skin and get rid of excessive oil. The antioxidants in tomatoes make them free radical fighters. Purchase organically grown tomatoes or grow your own to try one of these skin care techniques utilizing the tomato.

Turmeric ~ This is a spice that should be easy to find in your local grocery store. It is often used to prevent wrinkles due to its anti-allergic, antiseptic, antioxidant and nerve and blood vessel stimulating properties.

Vinegar ~ Vinegar has a multitude of uses. It restores the skin's natural pH balance. Do not apply it straight to your skin though. You'll want to dilute it with some water. Most often Apple Cider Vinegar is used.

Vitamin A ~ Vitamin A can be found in gelcaps in your local pharmacy. It is able to be absorbed by the skin and is a potent antioxidant. It is often used in anti-aging and healing products because it stimulates new cell growth.

Vitamin B3 ~ Vitamin B3 is also known as Niacin and has been shown as an effective treatment for acne. Some foods that contain Vitamin B3 and can be pureed and used as a mask are cranberries, tomatoes, soy sauce, summer squash and green peas.

Vitamin B5 ~ Vitamin B5 is also known as Pantothenic Acid and is used to increase the moisture content in skin and hair. Some foods that contain Vitamin B5 and can be pureed and used as a mask are avocado, cranberries, sunflower seeds, tomatoes, strawberries, yogurt, whole egg, winter squash and royal jelly.

Vitamin C ~ We all know that Vitamin C (also known as ascorbic acid) is great for the body, especially when we're feeling ill but did you know it is also great for the skin? When used on the skin it promotes healing, helps collagen development, can fight sun damage, is an antioxidant and may help reduce wrinkles and lines. Some foods that contain Vitamin C are oranges, peppers, grapefruit, peaches, papaya, grapes, apricots, broccoli, pineapple, tomatoes, strawberries, cranberries, kiwis, peas, sweet potatoes, lemons, mangos, tangerines, cantaloupe and honeydew melons.

Vitamin E ~ Every day we are bombarded with products that contain Vitamin E (Tocopherol). There is a reason for this. Vitamin E, like Vitamin A (Retinol), is an antioxidant as well as promoting cellular renewal. It is extremely healing and is an excellent ingredient in moisturizers and facial masks. It is often used as a preservative in some formulas. You can find Vitamin E in gel cap form (like the Vitamin A), which you will have to pierce with a pin or, to save yourself some time, you can also find it in liquid form.

Watermelon ~ Watermelons contain even more Lycopene than tomatoes do! See the entry on tomatoes for more information on Lycopene.

Wheat Germ ~ Wheat Germ has moisturizing, healing and exfoliating properties. It is one of the richest sources of vitamin E. The oil is very nourishing for dry skin and it also helps to reduce scarring. If you blend it with other oils it acts as a preservative to help them last longer because of its antioxidant properties. Some people think that Wheat Germ Oil smells like dead fish but it is an excellent source of Vitamins A, E and D. It is good to use for massage oils for the hands and feet and it has a very long shelf life.

Whole Wheat Flour ~ Whole Wheat Flour can help to slow down the aging process because it contains Vitamin E (which helps to bind environmental toxins), is anti-inflammatory, and promotes cell respiration. It also contains extra fiber which may provide additional exfoliating benefits, sloughing off dead skin cells.

Witch Hazel ~ Many of you may be familiar with Witch Hazel already but did you know it has toning, astringent, antiseptic and anti-inflammatory properties? It is soothing to irritated skin and doesn't dry it out. It also helps to prevent wrinkles by toning and refreshing the skin. Magickally Witch Hazel is used for protection and chastity.

Yarrow ~ Yarrow is astringent and anti-inflammatory. It is used often with acne prone skin. It can also be used as a sitz bath for those suffering from hemorrhoids. Yarrow is magickally associated with love, warding off negativity, repelling fear, courage, psychic powers, exorcism and protection from harm.

Yogurt ~ Yogurt has nourishing, cleansing and moisturizing properties. Just like a lot of the other items featured in this list, it is extremely useful not only in our diets but also in our beauty regimens. You want to make sure to always use plain, live yogurt which means that it contains live bacteria. The live bacterium in the yogurt is very helpful to acne-prone skin.

Bewitching Beauty by Starr Morgayne

Bewitching Beauty by Starr Morgayne

Companies

Ivy's Magickal Garden
P.O. Box 11496
Fort Wayne, Indiana 46858-1496
http://www.IvysMagickalGarden.com
~ Many of the products from these other companies can be found at this website also including products produced by Starr herself!

Burt's Bees, Inc.
P. O. Box 13489
Durham, NC 27709
http://www.burtsbees.com

Tom's of Maine
302 Lafayette Center
Kennebunk, ME 04043
http://www.tomsofmaine.com

THAYERS Natural Remedies
P.O. Box 56
Westport, Connecticut 06881-0056
http://www.thayers.com

Natracare LLC
14901 E. Hampden Avenue Suite 190
Aurora, CO 80014
http://www.natracare.com

GladRags
PO Box 12648
Portland, OR 97212
http://www.gladrags.com

Earth Mama Angel Baby
9866 SE Empire Court
Clackamas, OR 97015

http://www.earthmamaangelbaby.com

Our Natural Baby
240 Parkland Blvd.
Vermilion, Ohio 44089
http://www.ournaturalbaby.com

Simply Orange Juice Company
2659 Orange Avenue
Apopka, FL 32703
http://www.simplyorangejuice.com

Bewitching Beauty by Starr Morgayne

About the Author

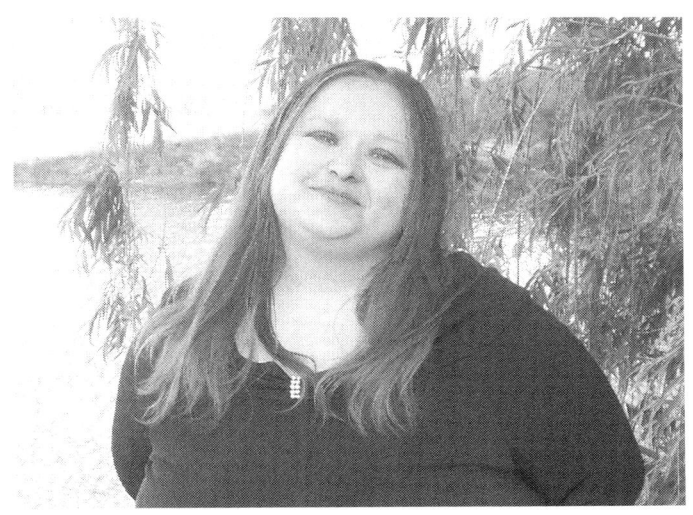

Starr Morgayne is in her mid thirties and has been studying herbs, alternative healing methods and alternative spirituality for more than 15 years. She has been the president of the Fort Wayne Pagan Alliance, local coordinator for her annual Pagan Pride Day for 2 years in a row (as well as helping coordinate previous years), a metaphysical shop owner and interviewed in her local newspaper along with the book Embracing the Darkness; Understanding Dark Subcultures to help dispel myths about Witches and Pagans. She has her 2nd degree in Usui Reiki and plans to go to college to get a degree in Naturopathy, Alternative Medicine and Herbalism. Her short stories have been published in several anthologies and she writes articles for a magazine tailored to esoteric and occult subjects.

She lives in Indiana with her four cats, three dogs, two ferrets, lots of fish and her loving family. In her spare time she enjoys writing, photography, crafting and gardening.

If you are interested in purchasing some of the skin care and other products that Starr makes they are available at www.IvysMagickalGarden.com.

Bewitching Beauty by Starr Morgayne

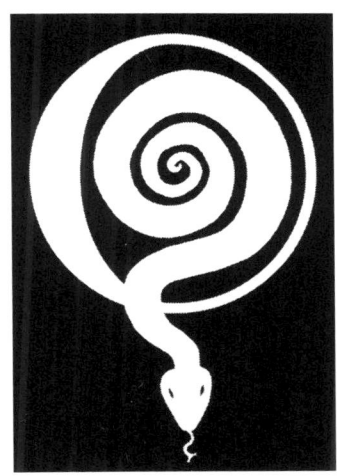

Dark Moon Press

P.O. Box 11496

Fort Wayne, Indiana 46858-1496

DarkMoon@darkmoonpress.com

www.darkmoonpress.com

Look for these and more titles on our website!

Bewitching Beauty by Starr Morgayne

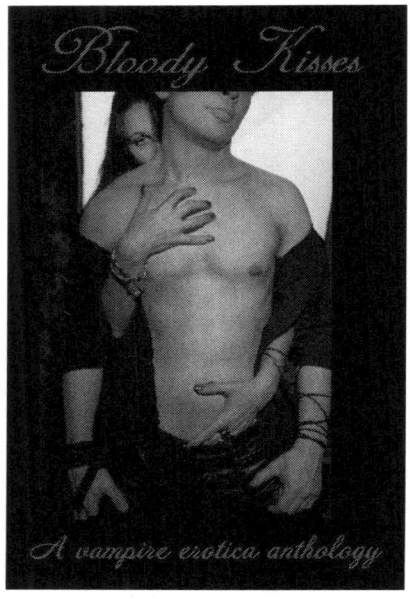

Bloody Kisses; A vampire erotica anthology

By Various Authors

A hot and steamy collection of blood soaked tales from authors such as Michelle Belanger, Raven Digitalis, Corvis Nocturnum, Mora Zoranokov and more!

WARNING: Adult Content

$17.95 USD, 192 pages, paperback

Originally released October 2007

ISBN: 9781451585872

Bewitching Beauty by Starr Morgayne

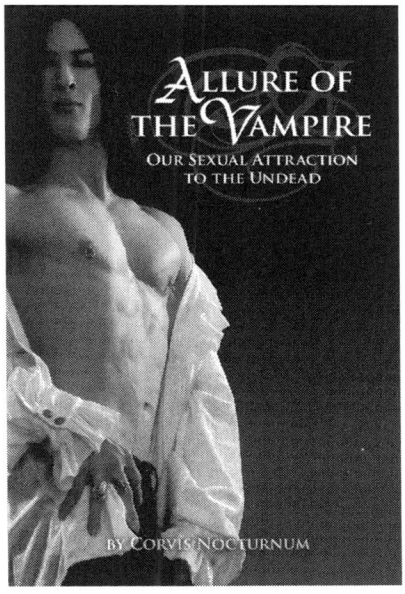

Allure of the Vampire:: Our Sexual Attraction to the Undead
By Corvis Nocturnum

The mere mention of vampires used to be enough to make people think of a nocturnal predator. But over the centuries the vampire has changed from monstrous villain to sexual object, for both men and women alike. *Allure of the Vampire* examines our intimate attraction to these beings in a detailed manner. Now, join occult author Corvis Nocturnum as he reveals the fascinating evolution of this icon as it has lured and enticed us in folklore, film and books from the days of ancient civilization to the living breathing inhabitants of our modern subculture, the vampire community.

$19.99 USD, 840 pages, paperback
August 2009

Bewitching Beauty by Starr Morgayne

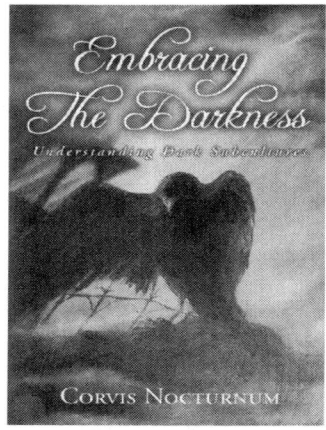

Embracing the Darkness
Understanding Dark Subcultures
By Corvis Nocturnum

The initial book of Dark Moon Press, written by author Corvis Nocturnum, which brings you an unprecedented collection of Satanists, vampires, modern primitives, dark pagans, and gothic artists, all speaking to you in their own words. These are people who have taken something most others find frightening or destructive, and woven it into amazing acts of creativity and spiritual vision.

Corvis himself is a dark artist and visionary, and so it is with the eye of a kindred spirit that he has sought these people out to share their stories with you.

$17.95 USD, 242 pages, paperback
May 2005
Cover art by Corvis Nocturnum
Cover design by Monolith Graphic

Bewitching Beauty by Starr Morgayne

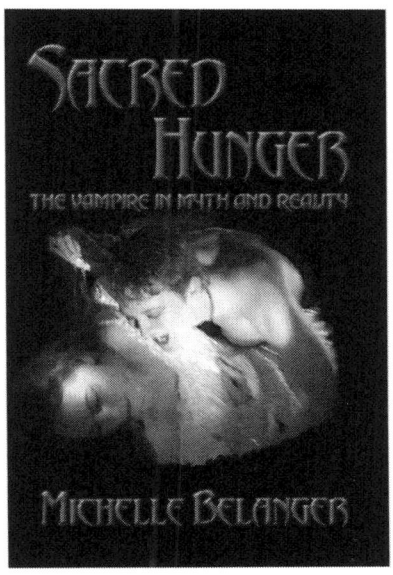

Sacred Hunger
By Michelle Belanger

Author Michelle Belanger has fascinated and informed readers about the vampire in folklore, fiction, and fact since the early 90s. Now enjoy all of Michelle's major essays on this fascinating topic, collected for the first time in one volume. Find out why author Bram Stoker wrote about vampires -- and what real-life psychic vampire inspired the figure of Dracula. Learn about the history and development of the modern community of real vampires. Explore the allure of the vampire in modern culture, and meet members of the vampire underground who have made this potent archetype a fundamental part of their lives...

$16.95 USD, 164 pages, paperback

Bewitching Beauty by Starr Morgayne

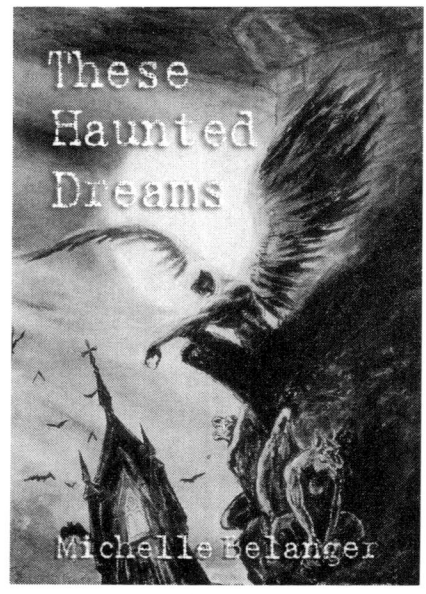

These Haunted Dreams
By Michelle Belanger

Dark, sensuous, and lyrical, the supernatural fiction of author Michelle Belanger has enchanted the readers of *Shadowdance*, *Necropolis*, and *Wicked Mystic* since 1991. Now, collected for the first time, enjoy the chilling and erotic tales of vampires, demon lovers, and ghostly visitations in *These Haunted Dreams*. A visionary artist sees too deeply into the secret life of one of his models. A businessman obsessed with time runs late for work and changes his life forever. A new homeowner discovers that his beloved residence is alive and has no intention of letting him leave. And many more...

$16.95 USD, 135 pages, paperback
Cover art by Corvis Nocturnum.

Made in the USA
Columbia, SC
20 January 2018